Advance Praise for *WHERE FAIRY TALES GO*

A powerful, moving story, beautifully written.
  Mike Lupica, New York Times #1 bestselling author, *Heat, Travel Team and Million-Dollar Throw*

A moving and beautifully written story of resilience, love, and faith.
  Donald T. Phillips, bestselling author, *Lincoln on Leadership*

This powerful narrative will grab you and not let go. I could not put the book down. Annette Ross's memoir chronicles a catastrophic medical error that profoundly affected her life with her husband Bill and their five daughters. Where Fairy Tales Go *reflects on medical ethics, faith, forgiveness and family. Above all it's a testament to the love that endures when two people have the courage to persevere in the face of tragedy.*
  Thomas H. Murray, author, *The Worth of a Child*

Annette Ross' story is a profound example of a family displaying courage and love in the face of undeserved calamity.
  Frank Roosevelt, co-author, *Understanding Capitalism*

Where Fairy Tales Go *is a compelling, candid reminder that when the world goes upside down, it's still possible to keep moving forward...a playbook for all of us about the power of love, the definition of home and the importance of family and friends.*
  Lee Woodruff, New York Times #1 bestselling author, *In an Instant*

Annette Ross' beautiful and deeply personal memoir invites you into her life through the most difficult of times and, in the end, you will see what bravery and faith look like.

Jacki Zehner, Chief Engagement Officer, Women Moving Millions and Former Partner and Managing Director, Goldman Sachs

Where Fairy Tales Go

Where Fairy Tales Go

A LOVE STORY

Annette Ross

Willow Street Press New York

ISBN-10: 0997831618
ISBN-13: 9780997831610
Library of Congress Control Number: 2016952134

Willow Street Press LLC Bronx NY
www.willowstreetpress.com

Printed in the United States of America

For Bill

and in loving memory of my father
William Palmer Fenwick Jr.

Prologue
Revisiting Home

~

May 2016

IT'S LIKE I'M CAUGHT BETWEEN two lives. There's the one I'm fully engaged in day-to-day; trying, with my husband Bill and our five daughters, to make sense of all that we lost. And there's the true-life fairy tale that once was, but exists now only in my memories. Those two realities collided recently, when we returned to Connecticut—to our best friends and our beloved neighborhood—but not to our old life.

Sixteen years have passed since the event that changed everything. Now, on the heels of my Dad's burial, we were gathering to celebrate a birthday and an impending birth. Living in California, we missed a great deal in the lives of our old friends back home, but we would not miss the birthday celebration for Bill's best friend George, or our friend Victoria's baby shower.

Our youngest, two-year-old Georgia, ran happily around the lawn in her red Minnie Mouse Mary Janes chasing after an enormous yellow lab and calling out, "Dottie! Come!" in her raspy, munchkin voice. We were staying with George and his wife Ann, who had been with us through so much. Looking over at the beautiful farmhouse next door, at what had once been our home, everything looked greener and brighter than I'd remembered, perhaps on account of the spring rain, or because my eyes had grown so accustomed to San Diego's myriad, muted shades of brown. I thought of how much our girls had grown: all teenagers (besides Georgia and Mia) with Natalie only a few weeks from her high-school graduation. I'd always pictured that milestone happening here, in New Canaan, with the friends she'd known since pre-school. Instead, on account of our peripatetic existence, she would be graduating 2,500 miles away, from the third high school she'd attended in four years.

I'll admit wholeheartedly (and with more than a twinge of guilt) that I'd hoped for a less challenging life. And on that lush spring afternoon, as I revisited the sweet, uncomplicated life we'd very nearly achieved, I wanted to hold on to this moment of perfection for just a little while longer.

The Delivery Room

January 2000

THE ANESTHESIOLOGIST ARRIVED IN A lousy mood.

It was after midnight. She looked disheveled and distracted. Her dirty-blond hair fell over her eyes. To diffuse the obvious tension, I began an anxious litany of questions to try and build rapport. I also needed to bolster my own courage. I asked how she was feeling. "Exhausted," she said, and mumbled something about having gone out with her new fiancé. The tone in her voice was unsettling. And she made it clear that she was not there for conversation. It was important to let her do her job, so I tried to talk myself down by nervously chatting with Bill. We were, after all, excitedly anticipating the birth of our second child. She brought with her a metal cart, instructed me to move to the end of the bed, and told me to "lean over the table." As she injected the needle into my lower back, my body jolted violently.

"Sit still," she yelled. But my movements had been involuntary. I let out a scream as a burning sensation ran down both legs simultaneously.

"What just happened?" Bill asked, looking serious. "Are you okay, Annette?" I took in a breath and thought, I'm still breathing. My thoughts were racing, I'm still breathing, I reminded myself. "I guess I am."

"How are you?" the doctor demanded, not hiding her annoyance.

"Something is not right," was all I could utter. The doctor's response: "You're being dramatic." She turned away from us.

Maybe so. I was in labor, my legs were on fire, and something had happened when she placed that needle in my back.

(Months later, when the nurses who'd been on duty that night were interviewed by our legal team, they said they'd heard me scream, but hadn't come in to see what had happened. They'd arrived later, to hold my legs during delivery. In her own deposition, the anesthesiologist used the word "histrionic" to describe my behavior.)

After the injection, and my violent jolt, the anesthesiologist left Bill and me alone in the room holding a bell—an actual bell—because the nurses' call button was disabled. (And *I* was histrionic?) I told myself, "Whatever that pain was, it's over. I'm okay." I looked again to Bill for reassurance. He held my hands in his and said calmly, "You're all right. You are. I promise." It was time to deliver.

Hospitals have those colorful diagrams with faces that range from wide-eyed smile to red-faced grimace to help children (and adults) describe their pain level. I thought about which one might describe mine—none seemed sufficient. What began as a mild twinge quickly escalated to the most intense, searing pain I have ever experienced. My legs were on fire. Strange sensations accompanied the burning. It felt like molten hot coils were wrapped around my legs and being squeezed tight, as if by a demon from Dante's *Inferno*. Any labor pain did not register, the only thing I felt was the screaming pain in my legs, as if they were crying from inside my body. But no one around me was listening.

My obstetrician—the one who had delivered our first daughter, Natalie, and with whom I had a trusting, established relationship—was away in Los Angeles when I went into labor. The OB covering for her was delayed in getting to the hospital, barely arriving in time to catch my baby.

Anna was born on January 5, 2000, at 2:39 a.m. She was perfect. Bill chose her name, because I had named Natalie. We couldn't wait to introduce our daughters to one another. But, it was not time to open the champagne. Something was definitely wrong. We told the on-call obstetrician that something very unusual had happened when I'd received the epidural—unlike anything I'd experienced with Natalie. "I'm sure it's fine," she said, with complete disregard. She appeared confident, so I told myself to focus on Anna. It was only a few hours until morning.

When we told the nurses about our concerns, they made notes and said, "Would you like more pain medication?"

"But there's something wrong," I insisted.

"We think you're anxious and need to relax," They left annoyed. We were getting nowhere.

Bill knew I was uneasy, but asked to meet his dad for breakfast. He probably needed some fresh air, but I didn't want him to leave. "Rest," he said. "Everything is going to be fine."

I was restless. What was wrong? I used the time to really focus on these strange sensations. Inside, my legs were alive, burning and pulsing; on the outside they felt heavy, I could not even wiggle a toe. I buzzed the nurse again to make my case. "Something's wrong. This didn't happen with my first delivery," I insisted. They offered me Valium to settle me down.

"The epidural is taking longer to wear off, but you're fine," they said. "You'll be up in no time."

"In *no* time," I thought. Yes. No time. Ever.

Eight hours after the epidural, my legs were numb. I couldn't feel the surface of my thighs. I scratched them hard, but nothing.

These were not my legs. They didn't feel as though they belonged to my body. Panicked, I phoned Bill. "Get back here," I shrieked. "Something terrible has happened!"

The nurses were ignoring me. Bill wasn't there. My baby was in the nursery. Not knowing what else to do, I prayed. The numbness travelled upward. My stomach started to lose sensation. My chest felt heavy. I prayed the most fervent prayer of my life. "Please don't let me die. Do not leave me." As I prayed the numbness in my chest and stomach retreated. My breath felt lighter. My legs remained as they were, but I was alive.

When my father visited later in the day, I explained what happened. He listened intently to my every word. And then, with tears in his eyes, he said, "God saved you."

"But Dad, it makes no sense. I'm still not walking," I was in anguish. "Has God saved my life but not my ability to walk?"

"We don't yet know what has happened with your legs," he said. "Take this minute by minute. You are alive, and where there's life, there's hope."

Sometimes he spoke with the wisdom and assurance of a priest. I was saved, but from what? Up to that very moment, I believed that God had answered all of my prayers exactly as I'd asked, whether it was something fairly inconsequential or getting accepted to the college of my dreams. I believed with my entire being that God existed, but this was the first time I truly needed to rely upon it being true. There had to be an answer. Bill was there. My father was there. The two people who loved me most in this world. Nothing bad could happen. Nothing that the doctors, or God, couldn't fix.

The day dragged on. The nurses and doctors *finally* began to suspect that something was actually wrong. The first series of MRI scans appeared unremarkable, that is to say fine, only they weren't fine. The seasoned doctors who read them missed the swelling that was invading my spinal cord. Had they seen it on the first run, they would have administered massive steroids to reduce the swelling, which might have salvaged some nerve conductivity. Hours passed, more doctors came in and scratched their heads, only to walk out again after my failed attempts to wiggle a toe. We waited. New doctors arrived. They started to whisper at the foot of my bed. "What is going on?" I demanded. "We don't know." They suspected a hematoma, but ruled it out. They sent me for more tests.

It was following my second three-hour MRI that they found something. A neurologist sat at the edge of my bed. "We know what's wrong," she gently said. That was the news we'd longed to hear. They'd identified the problem. Problems have solutions. Everything was going to be okay.

"You have swelling in your spine, transverse myelitis, and we need to move you to a hospital that can better care for your needs." Okay. I was ready to go. None of this sounded so terrible. Things were looking up.

We were given a choice of medical centers in Connecticut (where we lived) or New York City. We decided to go to Yale-New Haven Hospital. We struggled with whether Bill should join me in the ambulance or stay behind with Anna. There were many loving nurses to care for her, but she was our baby, just two days old. It felt wrong to leave her, and yet I needed Bill by my side. They transported us by ambulance. Bill would come back for Anna the next day. There was nothing to say as we left, only tears as we kissed Anna goodbye. It was a cold, quiet ride.

At Yale, a young resident whom we later referred to as "the Grim Reaper" arrived on the scene. His hair and his expression were black. He pulled out a marker and began to draw hieroglyphics on my cold legs. Bill stood beside me. "Do you know what has happened to you?" he asked, as if he was anxious to deliver the bad news. "Not fully," I replied. "You may never walk again," he said somberly.

"Do you know what a spinal cord injury is?" he asked. I didn't, but knew instinctively it wasn't good. He explained that the injury was not reversible, there was no going back, and it would be a long road. "That can't be true," I said, as I looked down at my legs. I started to touch them, rub them, almost hug them with my hands. They belonged to me, and I depended on them to move. I had no faith in this doctor's words. He didn't know me. I didn't believe for a moment that my body would betray me. I would heal.

I felt a flicker of hope each morning when the team of neurologists arrived at my bedside, armed with a coffee cups, clipboards, and pens. After a spinal cord injury, it's a positive sign if you can begin to move a toe—and the sooner the better. The residents would pull back my sheets and instruct me, "Wiggle your toes." I tried. I mean to say I really tried. My toes did not cooperate. My brain sent the signal. I could think the thought, but my body remained perfectly still. The young doctors jotted notes and looked at one another ominously. They'd never heard of an epidural causing paralysis before.

For three weeks, the same routine played out. "MOVE!" I demanded of myself. Nothing. Eventually, my internal voice would shift to a more plaintive, "please…just *move*." By the time I relinquished that morning's effort, my forehead would be covered in perspiration. It was a vastly different effort than going for a jog (something my body understood), but I was working just as hard to achieve a single, small motion.

After the residents left, their leader, Dr. Stephen Strittmatter, would often stay behind. A specialist with a lengthy list of impressive credentials, he was soft spoken and reserved, but also deeply compassionate. He spoke to me as a big brother would, and I felt that I was more than a diagnosis to him. I would eventually learn of his groundbreaking research, meet his family, and even attend a Christmas party he and his wife Jill hosted each year for the research team. Tests and trials are conducted far removed from patient care. He confided that having me there was a reminder that a real person would one day benefit from their sustained efforts. But right then, Dr. Strittmatter was out of the lab, and I needed him to explain to me, again and again, what had happened. I didn't get it. He described in simple, layman's terms what he saw on the films. He drew many pictures. He brought the MRI images to show me exactly where my spinal cord had narrowed.

"Here is your spinal cord as it runs down your back, do you see?" Yes, I saw it, and clearly. "Now, here's where it gets thin. Do you see how the cord narrows and looks slightly atrophied?" I had to look very closely, and yes, I could make out a slight narrowing of the black matter on the screen.

"*That's* my problem? You must be joking!" I thought that whatever was inhibiting my use of half my body would show up as something more obvious. But no. In the lower portion of my back, there was a place where the cord was a hair's-width thinner than the rest, and that was it. A nonevent if you ask me.

"There are no cures?" I pleaded. He was patient with me. I asked the same question every time I saw him, and each time he responded evenly, without the slightest hint of frustration. "We have made progress, and you might make some strides through therapy, but as of now, no, there are no cures." He looked to see if I understood him. I did; we did. Not knowing what else to say he squeezed my hand and left the room.

Most days, I cried. My inability to perform the simplest of instructions infuriated me. And yet, the doctors were always kind, sometimes offering a much-needed smile as they walked out.

There was nothing they could do to change things, beyond extending their humanity to a shattered woman. "They'll be good doctors," I thought. Dr. Strittmatter modeled genuine empathy for his team—the trait of an excellent physician. I believe it should be ranked more highly than any academic plaque on the wall.

Three weeks earlier, Bill and I had known exactly what lay ahead for us—life with a toddler and her newborn sister, a wonderful new home, a successful business, exceptional friends, and the excitement (and exhaustion) of balancing motherhood and graduate school. I'd picked out a light-blue checkered fabric for the chair in Anna's room. Her changing table was stocked with diapers, wipes, and pastel-colored onesies. The musical mobile hung quietly over the crib waiting to sing to its new arrival. We were all ready, including Natalie, who talked non-stop about her plans to care for her baby sister. We were truly blessed.

Now, my baby and I were both in diapers. I'd pictured rocking her in the early morning light, gazing out at the white pines beside our house. Instead, we shared a sterile, brightly lit hospital room. How was I going to care for her? Or for my little Natalie, waiting at home? The hospital made arrangements for Anna to come stay with me in the special-care-maternity wing. She arrived the day after my transfer. Natalie was being well looked after by my parents. Because I was being pumped full of steroids and other toxic chemicals, my breast milk was tainted, and Anna was not allowed to nurse. Once things improved and the doctors decreased my meds, I tried to pump—the nursing staff understood my desire to bond with Anna—but the milk never came in successfully. I felt such contempt for my body.

When she entered the world, Anna should have been center stage. Instead, she became the opening act and then the backdrop to the drama of my legs. During the day, a multitude of doctors and nurses cared for me, commanding much of my attention. It seemed that, any time I tried to focus on Anna, someone would enter the room to draw a vial of blood or administer a heparin shot. She was such a great baby. It was as though she understood at the tender age of 1 week old what we needed from her. She slept well, rarely cried, and sweetly cooed for anyone who gave her the attention she deserved.

The little time we had together—mother with her newborn baby girl—was late at night. When the hospital was quiet, I would hold Anna in the dark while Bill slept nearby on the couch. The tears spilled from my cheeks to hers. None of what happened seemed real. It was not supposed to be this way. Maybe it was the heavy medications, or my throbbing head, but I kept thinking I would awaken to realize that it had all been just a bad dream. Those were long nights. As Anna slept in my arms, I watched the shadows move slowly along the walls, and waited for morning.

Did God know what had happened? Where are you, God? I kept thinking He might come to me. Would He help? Maybe it was too much to ask. I needed to know, not from a doctor or nurse, but from Him, that everything was going to be all right. One day, a nurse named Nicole stopped in. She'd heard about my case, and said, matter of factly, "I have a message for you from God." Finally, I thought! She gave me a stuffed toy lamb for Anna, held my hands in hers, and quoted a passage from the Book of Jeremiah, "For I know the plans I have for you. Plans to prosper you and not to harm you, plans to give you hope and a future."

" I don't understand" I cried.

"I know, but you will," she said, with complete assurance. And, with that, a walking, breathing angel left my room.

Having Bill by my side each day and night was a constant reminder that I was not alone. His physical presence was a touchstone that enabled me to stay in the moment. My desire was to escape, but survival depended upon my ability to be still. Bill was the constant. He never left that hospital room until after I'd been there for weeks, and then only after my sister insisted that he take a night off. "Will you be okay if I leave?" he asked gently. I didn't know. He needed to see Natalie. My motherly instincts took over. "Yes, you should go." I said. "Tell her I love her." My sister had arrived the day before. She stayed up with me, and the night felt as long as the entire life I'd lived up to that point. I felt that I was having my first glimpse of death. When Bill returned the next day, I joked, "I'll bet the bed was comfy."

"No," he said. He'd barely slept. Together, we'd always slept perfectly, even when we woke to Natalie's cries. Bedtime was the part of day I most looked forward to, and our bed was a place of refuge for us. But Bill came back—back from the comfort of our bed at home to the hospital's bright lights and plastic sheets. "Thank God he came back," I thought.

Bill absorbed the shock and pain, and carried the burden of what I could not yet comprehend. In the hospital, he was my husband, trusted friend, and patient advocate. During hours of conversations with doctors who used terms we'd never heard of, Bill took notes, drew pictures—of the horse-tail-like bundle of nerves called the cauda equina—and tried to grasp how a cascade of unlikely events had led to my paralysis. We were both dumbfounded. He brought pillows from home that smelled of fresh laundry. While I held our sweet baby girl, my back against a soft pillow, I reminded myself, "I have a place to go after this."

He was at my side for every MRI scan—each of which took at least three hours. From inside that long tube, I could see him sitting patiently, earplugs firmly in place, holding tight to my pale, cold feet (even though he knew I couldn't feel them) as the synchronized knocking droned on. I didn't have to ask. He knew how much I needed him. And because he could handle it all—the smells, the sounds, the sterile environment, the constant interruptions, and the general pandemonium—I didn't collapse. Bill's unwavering devotion saved me. He couldn't cure me, but so early on in my shock and disbelief, he held me. God didn't show up. Or, maybe…He sent me His very best.

One week into our stay at Yale-New Haven, Natalie was allowed to visit. Her big blue eyes fixed on me. "Mama," she said. How I loved the sound of her little gerbil-like voice. I missed her so. She stood at the edge of the room, looking apprehensive as she clutching a stuffed toy intended for her baby sister. "You can come closer, honey," I called to her. She stayed put. "Natalie, come give Mama a hug," I beckoned. She reluctantly came closer and I held out my hand. The nurses brought Anna in. Natalie sat beside me in bed, and Anna was placed in the arms of her big sister.

I wept at the sight of these little girls together for the first time. My sorrow suffocated the joy. The moment stood silhouetted in my mind. It wasn't supposed to be this way. Natalie sensed something. There was no way to explain to this little girl—not yet even two years old—why her mother was so distraught.

Before this incomprehensible separation, Natalie and I had spent her every waking minute together, talking, cooking, walking in the yard. When the bleeding hearts bloomed in the courtyard, we'd made up stories about them. I sang to her as we sat on the swing, and we read *Moo, Baa, La La La!* over and over again, along with her other favorite picture books. Now, weeks into this new way of living, she looked shocked and frail...and something else as well. Her pediatrician came to see me in my hospital room. "I don't want you to worry, but Natalie's recent blood tests showed that she has a virus called TEC. She might need a transfusion to boost her platelet count." To be certain she didn't have cancer of the blood, Bill took her (along with his own dad) for a bone marrow test. Thankfully, the results were negative for leukemia. It was only the virus.

Each day, the doctor drew blood and closely watched her red blood cell count, which had dropped dangerously low. If her numbers continued to decline, she would have to be admitted into the hospital with me. Happily, her numbers began to improve incrementally over the next two weeks and she bounced back for a full recovery. How I longed to come home and resume our sweet daily routine. "Mommy is trying so hard, Nat, but it is not time. Not yet."

The nurses in special-care maternity were extraordinary. Two, especially—Nicole and Teri—cared for me like a dear friend. Teri was there to help me take my first post-injury shower. Before I undressed, I asked if she could stand me up. "If my feet touch the ground, I know I'll be able to feel them," I assured her.

"I'm not sure that is a good idea, Annette," she cautioned. But she helped me anyway. I looked down to see my feet on the

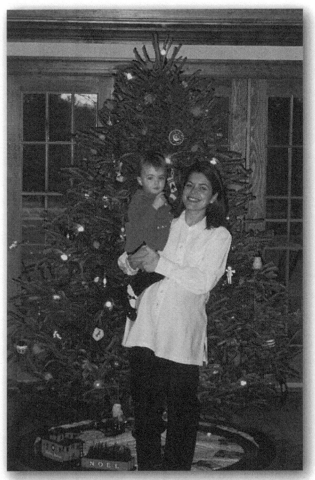

Christmastime with Natalie, about ten days before my injury. (1999)

ground. But I couldn't feel them. They looked flimsy, like Jell-O. Teri sat me back down. "Are you all right? Do you still want to shower?" The water was already on. I slumped over and wept. She hugged me until we were both soaked. Teri laughed and said, "Hey kiddo, should we get this done?"

"I am sorry I keep crying," I said. "Yes, I am ready to shower." The chair felt unsteady, but it was me shaking. I was weak. I did not have enough control through my core to bend over and shave or reach for the soap without losing my balance. I remembered the last shower I took before we left for the hospital. The championship game was on downstairs. Bill was enjoying the game with his cousin Tim when my water broke. As I climbed into bed in my grey flannel pajamas I heard a pop. "Bill," I called from the top of the stairs, "it's time to go!" Just a quick shower I thought. As the warm water ran down my body I prayed to Mary. "Watch over us Mary, watch over the baby, help us bring her safely into the world." All would be well. I hopped down the stairs with my little bag, kissed Mom and Dad (who came quickly to watch Natalie) and we headed into the night.

I do not want to remember, I thought. The water mixed with my tears until Teri turned it off. My constant crying didn't dissuade either nurse, as they saw me through each new assault on my body. A part of me wanted to scream, but my upbringing taught me to be polite. Besides I liked them. Even as they extracted quart after quart of blood, I wanted to smile and say "thank you." I have never liked having my blood drawn. Unfortunately, small veins are my trademark. After three jabs a phlebotomist was called in. "Your veins keep collapsing," she complained. "They make poor IV channels." Not much I could do about that. Still, I felt somehow inadequate. I wanted so much to be an exemplary patient; to be cheerful and responsive. But, it was hard to be nice; the high doses of steroids disoriented me. I became agitated, even toward the sweet, smiling people who were helping me. After days of being plugged in, I attempted to pull out the tubes that hovered above me. A nurse I didn't yet know entered the scene of my crime. (One is never alone in the hospital except for weekends and late at night.)

"What're you doing?" she asked, coyly. Busted.

"I cannot take being attached to this drip thing any longer," I sobbed.

"Well, you're not allowed to do this," she continued.

"Not *allowed*," I thought, suddenly seeing the nurse as my enemy. But I asked as calmly as possible, "*Please*, can you remove my IV and give me oral medications instead?" She left the room.

Nicole and Teri came to my rescue. "Honey, you do need a break. Your arms need a break. I've checked with the doctor, and we'll unhook these for the rest of the day" I was free. Scratched, bruised, and bloody, my arms looked as if I'd been attacked by wild animals. Being free and unhindered offered a moment's peace. I ran my fingers over the needle marks and thought, this can't be the way to heal.

Family and friends came to see me. I tried to greet everyone who entered with a smile (even if I shed a few tears during their visit). They mostly looked as though they were seeing a ghost. No one really knew what to say. "You look better than we thought you would," a friend said. Her honesty was not lost on me. I wanted to know what I looked like to the outside world. The steroids gave me a moon face, and my legs had lost their definition. It didn't take long for them to become flesh hanging over bone. I tried not to look at them, or at myself. It was better to stay positive, and pour that positivity toward moving my toe, or my legs, or going to the bathroom. Time was still on my side. Should I establish a neurological connection, the odds of my walking again greatly increased. As each new visitor arrived, we experienced their shock together, and I relived my horror. Yet they all reinforced my hope that soon I would be up and back home with our girls.

My brain was in constant hyper drive. If thinking were an Olympic sport, I might have won the gold. I started to consider the "what ifs." What if…my regular obstetrician hadn't been on vacation the night of Anna's birth? She was a witness to my first epidural with Natalie. She would not have allowed me to have one without her being present. I'd met her through the woman we bought our first house from in New Canaan. Had we not bought that house, would I have delivered at a different hospital? With a different outcome? Was I destined to end up in a wheelchair no matter what? Had we never left Chicago, where Bill and I met, would I have been hit by a car instead? Oddly enough, thinking through other "what if" scenarios made me feel better, because it allowed me to envision a world in which I might still be able to walk. When my trusted obstetrician came to visit, she called my mental machinations "magical thinking."

"You're more fortunate than you think right now," she said. "You *will* go home. This is not the end for you." But, it was the end. It was the end of many things.

Mom and Dad raised me to believe the intercession of the Saints can heal us. My father was as close to a living saint as anyone I have ever known, but was he close enough? Did he possess that kind of authority? He and Mom drove to the National Shrine of Padre Pio in Pennsylvania, bringing with them a pair of my pants that they touched to a relic of the Saint at the church's altar. When they returned, I cried tears full of hope, still believing that I might escape this fate. Maybe once I pulled the pants over my quiet legs something would happen. But nothing did (at least not in that instant). The efforts Mom and Dad made to heal me *did* bring about healing. Not in a way that allowed me to sprint for the door, but by momentarily lifting my heavy heart. And, days before my departure for rehab, just as Dad predicted, I was able to draw my right knee slightly toward my chest with my hip flexor. It was exhilarating. Everyone came in to cheer. My left leg lay dormant, but any movement can be built upon.

I derived energy from this positive development, and used it in attempts to regain my dignity and my ability to use the bathroom on my own. Maybe if I sat on the toilet and prayed something would happen. The nurses turned the water on and left the room to help me focus. I recited the same prayer over and over again. I pushed on my bladder. Nothing happened. "Just be patient," the nurse said when she came in to check on me. Three hours passed. All I had to show for my effort was a bright red ring on my buttocks. As I sat stared at the blank bathroom wall as if it would reveal some secret, a Biblical passage crept into my mind. "My grace is sufficient for you." The very words said to the Apostle Paul when he asked for the thorn to be removed from his side. It was not a voice from the heavens, but one from within the crevices of my own brain. I couldn't shake it. Had I taken it as a sign, I would have called it quits on my sit in a lot earlier. I had been confusing prayer with my own will. It became evident that I was not going to walk out of Yale hospital.

Dr. Strittmatter, Nurse Nicole, and Nurse Teri all became my dear friends, and remain so even to this day. They shared with me some of the most brutal, frustrating, and bewildering weeks of my life. Days spent negotiating bed pans and enduring urinary tract infections. Nights spent holding my newborn baby while tears streamed down my face. I felt that I was at war, with my own body, and with life itself for letting me fall. The team at Yale took this beaten-down soldier and lifted her up. They shielded me, grieved with me, and cried with me. There was not much I could offer in return, except for my heartfelt thanks. Those were weeks I soon wanted to forget, except for the moments where my suffering was met with human tenderness. I was the grateful recipient of their love. And, as the swelling in my spinal cord decreased, my legs were healing. There was more to work with than we'd once thought.

The even greater achievement was the dramatic shift in my emotional state. My hospital stay began in total despair; the life I envisioned as a wife and mother destroyed by a doctor's needle. But, I left feeling lighter—not physically—but with the lightness that comes from a burden shared. Even more than the doctors, the nurses reminded me of who I was, and that my purpose, whatever it might be, could be achieved regardless of my ability to walk.

Rehab

~

WE LEFT YALE-NEW HAVEN ON Bill's birthday, January 20, 2000. His mom made sure we had cake to mark the occasion. We headed north to a rehabilitation facility in Wallingford, Connecticut, cake in hand, but without our precious daughters. We were ready to do whatever was necessary to get me back home.

"You must learn to adapt to life in a wheelchair," explained the rehab doctor.

I had zero interest in that. "What about walking again?" I asked.

"The therapists will work with your legs, but the focus will be occupational therapy." And then he added, "Don't you want to be able to care for your baby?" No! I thought. Not like *this*!

If hospitals are dreary, rehab facilities are worse. Occupational therapy? I wasn't even sure what that meant. But I was to be institutionalized until I could master four skills: bladder catheterization, to enable me to urinate; sliding-board transfer, from bed to chair, chair to car, etc.; pressure-release lifts, to build triceps-muscle strength that would allow my lower body to hover, periodically, over my seat; and "wheelchair-level care" of my newborn (whatever that meant).

It seemed ludicrous that an unmarried 22-year-old therapist was explaining to me—a mother of two—how to diaper my child. And demeaning to be schooled in tasks as seemingly simple as pulling eggs from the fridge. If it had not actually been happening to me, it might have made for a funny *Saturday Night Live* sketch but, in truth, it was hard work. Everything that once was beautiful had turned grotesque. The thought of having to hold Anna within this bulky, cumbersome wheelchair made me recoil. I hated all of it. The worst part of rehab was "relearning" tasks I'd had mastery of when I could walk.

As my therapists worked, I noticed the effortlessness of their movements. It seemed they were mocking me. Their agility felt like a personal affront to my defective body. Was it me, or were their instructions all tinged with a note of condescension? "You can do this, Annette!" sounded like a middle-school cheerleader patronizing me as I attempted to diaper a baby doll on the edge of a bed.

"Yes, of course I can *do* this." I thought, wrapping a diaper around a doll. "I just cannot do *this*," as I looked down at myself.

At some point each day, I cried. Maybe it was hormonal or I hoped so because I cried, a lot. Our girls were both at home and, if my leg function was not going to improve, it seemed purposeless to stay in rehab any longer. We called a meeting with the physiatrist (a physician specializing in physical medicine and rehabilitation).

"What does Annette need to do so I can bring her home?" Bill asked. According to the doctor, I'd mastered everything but the catheter. That damn catheter was giving me so many problems. I couldn't locate my urethra, even with a mirror. (Before this happened, I hadn't even known I had one.) Whenever I got close to the mark, I would jab myself with this little plastic tube, leaving a fairly sensitive part of my body bruised and bloody. "What if I just can't do that?" I asked, exasperated.

The doctor was clear from the start and stated once again, "If you can't catheterize, then you can't leave."

Bill suggested a brilliant idea. "What if I learn to catheterize her?" The doctor considered that an acceptable solution. The nurses taught Bill how to find my urethra—he had the benefit of being able to see it, but even he missed the first few times. It is very small! Thankfully, he was not easily intimidated. Once he got it, he did it brilliantly. He proved more careful than anyone at the rehab center. We were on our way home within a week.

Bill administered my heparin shots, saw to my bowel routine and, of course, inserted the daily intermittent catheter. I wondered how all this would affect our marriage in the long run, but for now we were singularly focused on being back at home with our sweet girls. The rest would have to wait, including his work. For a man running his own business, this wasn't ideal. We had help, but the lion's share of my care fell to Bill. He said he wanted it that way, that he did not want to desert me. And because he offered, I did not have to ask. In truth I wanted no one else to witness what was happening, it was so intensely personal that he was the only one I could allow in.

But it left him with little time to work, and almost none for him to decompress. He had a couple of buddies who offered him a reprieve once in a while, but his absences stressed me. He rarely got out, not for a game, not for a beer, not for much of anything. In his high school yearbook, rather than borrow a quote from an author or politician, Bill had made up his own: "Life is a war, and every day is a battle." I'd always wondered at its meaning. (Had my school had senior quotes, I'd have chosen a line from a Beatles song like, "All you need is love.")

Once something terrible happens, everyone around you grasps for the silver lining as they struggle to help you, and also make sense of it for themselves. People have a need for this. But Bill and I had been very close and extremely happy before my injury. Did we need to be closer? Did he need to become my constant bathroom companion? We found the silver linings of our situation to be too few. Here's what I learned—that the depth of our incredible relationship, as lovely as it is, would have been fine as it was. It had not needed a proverbial kick in the teeth. That truth was hard to reconcile. Soon, Bill's mantra would become our reality—we *were* at war.

Orphaned and Adopted

~

PRIOR TO THE EVENTS OF January 2000, my life had not been without its ups and downs. But I'd always held tightly to my hopes and dreams. Life for me began in Chicago, at an orphanage run by the Sisters of Notre Dame. The very first hands to hold me, feed me, swaddle me were those of the Sisters. It has always bothered me to think that I didn't leave the hospital with parents who had anxiously planned for my arrival. The balloons, flowers, and excitement were missing from the picture. To comfort myself, I pictured the nuns holding me tenderly, and humming hymns while I drifted off to sleep.

My biological mother had not embraced her pregnancy, I learned later, referring to me as "a tumor growing inside of her." She left me behind. Eventually, I would have a chance to meet the woman who gave me up, to learn more about her, and to recognize her as beautiful and fragile, with a sensitive soul.

The parents who eventually adopted me fostered children through Catholic Charities. No longer a transient visitor, I belonged to someone, and not just someone, but to a big family. In all, Betty and Bill Fenwick would adopt four of us, in addition to having five biological kids. My brother Bruce said the family took to me right away. You might even say they spoiled me. Whatever time I spent in a crib at the convent was made up for with this new family of people to hold me.

We lived in Harvey, Illinois, just south of the city, in a concrete structure with a very large porch. I have little recollection of the inside, except that the Dad installed a water fountain to keep us from using too many cups. I vividly remember the backyard, where he built a bridge where my brother Marty and I would play, pretending to inhabit two worlds, one on either side. We eventually moved farther south, putting more distance between ourselves and Chicago's city limits after someone—we never learned who—smashed a brick through our front window. The new house was larger, the neighborhood safer. The fenced-in backyard was a perfect square with a pear tree in the very center. It was there that I began planning my future, in all its splendor.

When I was still a toddler, I was diagnosed with hip dysplasia and fitted with a brace. This metal-and-plastic contraption became a permanent part of my attire, day and night, for years. When I sat on the floor, my legs were stretched out to either side of my body. (It should have been the beginnings of a successful cheerleading career.) I learned to walk in that brace, and could even navigate a full flight of stairs. Once the brace was removed for good (at age three), I rarely thought much about it until after

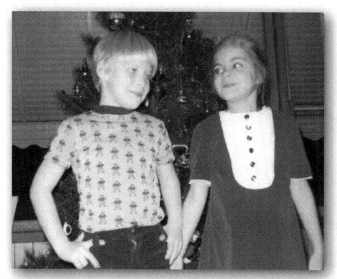

With my brother Marty.

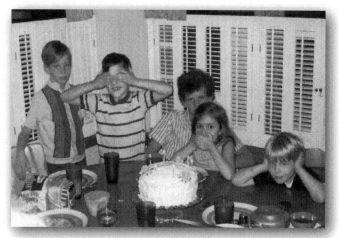

With four of my brothers. All the adopted kids together.

I'd lost the use of my legs…a curious coincidence.) All those years in braces caused my feet to turn out like a duck's. It took some doing, but we corrected it—my first bout with "physical therapy" which never meant going to a facility, but my work—with my body. My dad reminded me often to focus on how I walked and ran, and when I did my gait corrected itself, but it took the constant repetition, patience and sheer will. After that, I started to run, and became the fastest girl in my class. This skill would serve me well years later, working at the Chicago Board of Trade…the job that would lead me to Bill!

My parents didn't tell my brothers and me that we were adopted until 1976, when I was nine years old. They may never have—at least not then—if my school teacher hadn't chosen to blurt out, "You're adopted, didn't you know?" in front of my entire class. I'd run straight home and, with tears running down my face, asked my Mom if I was, indeed, adopted.

"Why do you ask?"

"The teacher said so."

Over the next several hours, she repeatedly asked, "What's wrong with being adopted?"

Each time I patiently replied, "Nothing's wrong with it, as long as I am not."

We played this strange little game until Dad came home. The thought of being adopted repelled me so much, I felt my worst fears realized. Who did I belong to? What did my real parents look like? Were they looking for me? Had I not been worth fighting for? These questions made me feel separate and alone. My Mom refused to quell my fears (she was good at that), and when Dad finally arrived, they told all four of us that, yes, we'd been adopted. My immediate response was tears. My brothers, Marty, Drew, and Gale, seemed to move on more quickly, shifting their focus to, "What's for dinner?"

My own list of questions was inexhaustible, and held me in a trance. But the crucial question was "Why?" My parents came up to my room later to reassure me. "Ann, we chose you. You're special. The day we brought you home was one of our happiest." I believed they loved me. I just didn't want to be adopted. That night, my brother Drew checked in on me. "Do you think you'll ever look for your biological parents?" I gave him an emphatic "No way. Never." He said he wanted to find his. It felt too disloyal to even consider. But years later, *I* was the one whose curiosity drove me to find my birth mother. Had I bonded with my adoptive Mom, it might not have felt necessary. I never thought to look for my biological father because there could be no better father than the one I grew up with. I knew I belonged to him. I put the thought of looking on hold for years. After Bill and I married, it was time. By then, I believed I could handle whatever my search might reveal.

When I myself became a mother, it helped clarify some of my feelings about being given up. Having watched my babies take their first breath, I knew instantly that there was nothing I would not do for them. To give them up would be like losing a part of my body. And yet I also understood, from an adult's perspective, that there are situations in which such a painful choice might be the most selfless decision a parent can make. But a child cannot fathom such complexities, and the sense of abandonment leaves a permanent scar. At least it did for me.

My childhood desperation for a fairy-tale ending—in which my birth parents heroically overcame obstacles to find me and care for me, and for them to have felt that I had been worth fighting for—is not unlike the recurring dream of my adult life: to walk again.

Years before my parents broke the adoption news, I had intermittently felt an incredible void. The first time it morphed into actual terror, I was five-years-old. While playing upstairs alone, I suddenly found it hard to breathe, and all that was familiar in my comfortable bedroom turned hostile. Gripped with steady fear, normal things began to seem unreal. I experienced a total absence of being. Rushing to the bathroom, I looked at myself in the mirror for what seemed like a very long time. "Breathe, Annette. You're here. You're okay." But the image I sought was beyond my face. I was searching for God—for something or someone—to find me. To my mind, God had been present only minutes earlier. (Those were the days when my definitions for "God" and "magic" were interchangeable.) Finally, a sense of relief spilled over my body, my breathing slowed, and the dread receded like waves from the shore. God seemed to hear my prayer. That fundamental, simple faith was enough to anchor me. Or, maybe I had helped myself out of that unknown place. Yet even today, so many years later, I take comfort in the image of God's large and powerful hand picking me up and taking me out of harm's way.

I never told Mom or Dad about that incident. But being alone was never the same for me after that, and anxiety would strike me during times of stress or heightened emotion, whether happy or sad. As I grew older, I prayed to understand the emptiness inside me. I thought again of the verse in Corinthians, about Paul and the thorn in his side. I had one as well. And if God chose not to remove it, maybe I needed to pray for grace. (A realization that was not lost on me in later life.) This particular passage uniquely united the pieces of my broken spirit and became a central theme throughout my life. The reluctant apostle who lost his eyesight only to have it fully restored was never fully healed. God left something for Paul to suffer, something to keep him humble? The Bible never states exactly what his thorn was, some scholars suggest it was anxiety, and I choose to align with them as it makes Paul's trials mirror those of my own. Paul asked God three times to remove his affliction, but God allowed it. I felt sorry for Paul and never understood why God chose not to heal him.

A few years later—not long after learning the news of my adoption—I decided to run away. My parents were having a party, and from upstairs, I could hear the hum of voices. Even though I'd been encouraged to join the festivities, I decided that no one really wanted me there. I had no plan. I only knew that I did not belong there. Pajamas and a toothbrush took up most of my tiny green-plastic suitcase. No one heard me leave. They were all too busy having fun, and by the time they did figure out I was gone, it would be too late. I headed down the long dark sidewalk. The street was quiet. I stood contemplating my next move. Would they be upset if I left for good? Surely my Dad would worry. I imagined them running around the neighborhood trying to find me, and suddenly my throat felt tight. I held my suitcase and squeezed back the tears. It wasn't them, it was *me*. I felt inadequate, and sometimes, but not always, when everyone was together laughing and having fun, I felt I did not belong there. But I wanted them to want me. It was about then that I realized that I was standing in front of the neighbor's house whose son once hit me with a stick as I rode past on my bike. Before he could have another chance, I made a run for home. I opened the door and slipped up the back stairs to my room. No one ever even knew I had left.

The same crippling fear overtook me again the night I was crowned homecoming queen of my high school class of 1985. Dad whispered over my shoulder, "I knew it would be you." I stepped forward, careful not to trip. As the tiara was placed on my head, tears of joy streamed down my face. But after posing for photos and heading home to change out of my long dress before celebrating with my friends, I became motionless. Suddenly, I felt that something terrible was going to happen.

"Dad, come in here," I called out nervously.

"What's wrong, Ann?" he asked. Mom stood behind him. She cared that I was upset, and yet she hadn't come to see me crowned. Why?

My breathing grew rapid and shallow, my heart pounded inside my rib cage. The room wasn't really there. We were no longer in our home.

"What's wrong, Ann?" he asked again. "If you tell me, I can help you."

I stood silently; unable to move, sit, or take a step forward. My father took my hand and led me to a chair. I sat down, and the room came back into focus.

There were times when I would become so afraid that it felt as if everything was closing in around me. And yet, I couldn't identify the source of my fear. It was like being chased by an invisible monster where there was no escape. "What's wrong with me, Dad?"

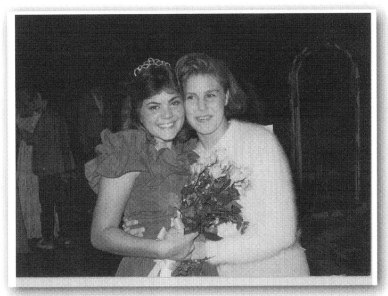

With my friend Amanda the night I was
crowned homecoming queen. (1985)

"We are all afraid," he said, "but strong when we are together."
And then he quoted a poem by Eve Merriam as he held my hand:

Frightened, you are my only friend.
And frightened, we are everyone.
Someone must make a stand.
Coward, take my coward's hand.

Mom and Dad

~

My mom and dad were complete opposites, at least to my mind. I often wondered how they stayed together for nearly sixty years. Because I love a love story, I asked them often to tell me about how they met. They both worked at a J.C. Penney department store on 154th street in Harvey, Illinois. Dad's mother worked there, too, as a seamstress, and it was she who introduced them to one another. Dad thought Betty was beautiful. Her given name was Mary Elizabeth. To be playful, and because she was just barely over 5 feet, Dad called her "Shorty," which irritated her. And yet, not so much that she didn't say yes to a first date. They courted, fell in love, and he proposed in front of the one landmark that survived the city's great fire, the Chicago Water Tower. It was indestructible, and so were they. On August 6, 1949 they married, both were 21-years-old. On one anniversary he had a picture of the water tower framed for her. Each time I went down Michigan Avenue I made a point to stop there and imagine the two of them in their excitement. They were so young and, like all of us who make that brave step to bind our lives to another, they knew nothing of what lay ahead. Whenever they talked of their early years together, they both smiled at the memories. They were in love and unabashed about showing it; they even kissed in front of us, all of the time. That was when I learned that what happens between two people is a mystery to those on the outside. Even though I lived with them, I could not understand their relationship as husband and wife. They were happy together, and later I realized it was not for me to understand.

As parents, they inhabited a hierarchical world of black and white. Things were either right or wrong, and not up for discussion. You were either part of the solution or part of the problem. If you got in trouble, the "why" didn't matter: you were reprimanded and given a penalty. Life consisted of routines and schedules: dinners together as a family when Dad got home, Mass every Sunday, and chores. I suspect that such rules have to be established when you have nine children, foster even more kids, and run a babysitting service all in one house. Being deeply religious, our parents established clear rules for us. They wanted us to be honest, respectful and hard-working.

Mom and Dad manifested their spiritual devotions differently. Dad was a convert to Catholicism. His Protestant background gave him a broader context from which to interpret the Bible. He always carried with him a small, black-leather copy of the *New Testament* in which he made copious notes and underlined his favorite passages. He read it so often that he eventually needed a rubber band to hold the book together. He was so moved by certain passages that he would copy them onto index cards when he thought I could use inspiration. Love notes from my Dad. "For God so loved the world that he sent his only Son," was arguably his favorite. I didn't understand the meaning. "Annette, it means that God loves you and you are special." To his way of thinking, offering a biblical passage to fix the problems of my life was a concrete solution. "We can all be healed," he would say. And to some degree, I believed it.

Educated in strict Catholic schools, Mom learned her Catechism, but her spiritual practice was restricted to obedience to the dogma and traditions of the Church, period. The overall message of love was absent. Good deeds mattered and were done, but rarely with loving intentions.

For Mom, Dad was her whole life, her sole happiness, and a window on the outside world. She never went out without him...ever. Never met a friend for lunch or coffee. She remained inside, doors shut, windows closed, curtains drawn. Only when Dad was home did she truly come to life. If there was a dispute between any of us and Mom, she had only to take it to the court of Dad, and no one but Mom would get the verdict they wanted.

I wish she'd given the rest of us a chance, but her fear that we might find out she was human prevented any of us from being especially close to her. Irish to the core, Mom dealt more easily with meat and potatoes than with emotions (her own or ours).

My oldest brother Buzz summed Mom up best when he said, "Mom is like sand in soup. Just don't stir it up."

Somehow, Mom could handle the disorder of a house filled with children, including at least four additional kids each day through her babysitting business. She ran a tight ship, maintaining feeding schedules, nap times, and diaper changes (we kids all helped in that department). Yet, she never learned to drive. We were told that she'd gone for the driver's test when she was in her twenties, but something happened, and she never got behind the wheel again. Later, she claimed that we were the real reason, and Dad protected her fiercely. "Mom's busy taking care of you guys, that's why she doesn't drive." Like my Mom, I loathe driving. But I don't blame my girls for it. I try to take ownership of my fears, in part because I remember the guilt I felt when my own mother didn't.

Mom was talented, but not gifted. A very competent seamstress, she made pantsuits and dresses for herself, my sister, and me. Patti and I even modeled some in local fashion shows. The ladies from Church fawned over her creations. Some of her hobbies provided supplemental income. She set up a dog-grooming table in the basement, and also bred poodles. It's so impressive to me now, but I didn't recognize it at the time.

Mom and I never had an easy relationship. She lacked my father's wisdom or his deep, constant love. And there was a sadness about her. I don't think she desired so many children but, being

Catholic, she wanted to do the right thing, and to follow Dad. With her sixth pregnancy—a stillborn boy, her uterus ruptured. There would be no more babies. It was then that she and Dad began taking in fosters and eventually adopted four of us. Whether it was my Catholic upbringing or my desire to make them proud, I, like my mother, have always wanted to do the right thing, even if my heart did not follow my sense of obligation. Maybe the problem was that I too often thought I knew what the right thing was, not realizing there were alternatives. It was always survival. But, did I foster my Dad's loving spirit?

As I observed Mom with the foster children, it struck me that one can do something good, but not really want to do it. So many children passed through the doors of our home. She took them in—both my parents did—but it was Mom who fed and clothed them. And yet, she rarely talked to them. I never remember her asking them directly how they were doing. I never recall her embracing these scared little children. She did not have that to offer—only bed space.

Certain kids stood out, like Tommy, who arrived with cigarette burns on his feet. Mom and Dad discussed adopting him—fearing for his future—but our house was already busting with kids. The caseworkers eventually took him back to the family where he was abused, and we never saw him again. Children like Tommy became the backdrop of my growing-up years. I have always wondered what became of them but, as a child myself, I was able to compartmentalize my concern for their circumstances.

How could their suffering be right in front of me, and yet worlds away? This may be a flaw in human nature, or my own personal flaw. We are all diminished or strengthened by what happens to others, but it's easier to put aside the pain when it was not your own to bear. The plight of the foster children became make-believe to me. I wanted no less for them than I did for myself, but I also wanted nothing to penetrate the idealized world I longed for. My happy life awaited, far from the sorrow, the mess, and the relentless noise of home.

What made Mom happy were *things*. Dad could never afford fancy gifts so, to make up for it, he drove her to weekend garage sales where she happily sought out what she considered real treasures. She would return home and boast, "Annette, look! A spoon with a mother-of-pearl handle! You will not believe what I paid for it! It cost nothing!" This was the most excited I ever saw her. She ended up with a lot of spoons, stacks of china plates (although never a complete set), and hundreds of sewing patterns that she never got around to making.

Because of Mom's acquisitive nature, and in part because of our family's sheer numbers, the house was filled with clutter. Underneath the stairwell, Mom stored thousands of magazines. You could find issues of *National Geographic* spanning the '50s, '60s, and '70s, if you looked long enough. Every drawer and cabinet was stuffed with mysterious items that, once opened, proved impossible to close. In the basement, boxes were stacked to the ceiling. I imagined their contents to include worn-out shoes, old

Halloween masks, and the odd mouse carcass. I never knew for sure, but since they also presented a perfect hiding place from which someone could jump out, I held my breath and ran for it each time I was sent downstairs to procure a can of green beans.

To my Mom's way of thinking, the hours I spent daydreaming were a waste of time. She could not share in the fantasies of my future happiness. She wasn't capable of being happy for another person. Were she able to imagine my dreams coming true, that might somehow diminish her own. My final years at home were one long argument with her. Being the youngest of nine, I was one of only two kids still living under our parents' roof. My brother Marty was gone most of the time, and Dad was working a job that kept him away during the week. When Dad would come home on weekends, tired and stressed, Mom made sure to involve him in all our disagreements. "Apologize to your mother!" he would say, once she filled him in. I'd try to argue my point, seeking justice in his eyes, but he would only grow more irate. Eventually, I would retreat. It was too painful to see him get so upset. Once we were all out of the house, Mom seemed happier. An occasional comment could send us back into battle, but she had mostly mellowed.

My Hoped-for Life

~~

EVERYONE IN THE FAMILY WAS expected to work. My first job (outside of my babysitting duties at home) was at the local arcade, during the summer between seventh and eighth grades. I mopped floors and exchanged quarters for tokens so that kids could ride the bumper cars, shoot down the giant slide on potato sacks, or use the batting cages. The job was ten hours each Saturday and Sunday but with many friends coming by, and an odd assortment of interesting characters hanging around, it was the perfect place for a middle schooler. My next job, at Burger King, required me to wear an odious tight brown polyester uniform, complete with hair net and brown plastic shoes—an absolute repellent to teen-age boys. My manager always put me on broiler duty; hot work, but not difficult, and better than being out front where friends could see me. Later, as a hostess at Bennigan's, I underwent a fashion metamorphosis. The requisite cotton polo shirt and kha-ki skirt transformed me; at last I was comfortable. On weekends I worked 9-to-5 at a boutique called Rosalie's then ran across the street to work the 6-to-2-a.m. shift at Bennigan's. I wasn't saving much money—not enough for college—but I was putting in the effort to pursue my dream of an idyllic life.

I remember hearing Mom and Dad argue about my college prospects. I heard Dad say, "Betty, she's smart and she wants to go." Mom did not agree, but relented. Dad helped me get financial aid and loans, and my best friend and I headed off to Illinois State University. The academics were fine; the classes interesting. I even studied agriculture, which made sense when you're living amongst the cornfields of Normal, Illinois. (I didn't think I would ever plant crops, but wanted to understand how food made it to the grocery store.)

But there was a problem: me. My anxiety prevented me from being comfortable there. During long, sleepless nights, I would call Dad. "I'm so scared. There's nothing out here…only corn." His voice made me feel safe. The conversation would shift away from scary things, to the birds in the backyard, or to the existence of God. Sometimes, I would fall asleep with the phone in my hand. A few times, we were still talking when the sun came up. After the first semester, I came home, and my anxiety vanished. Later Dad said, "Annette, it wasn't the open fields. A person can be happy anywhere. Happiness comes from within."

After my failed semester, I went back to Bennigan's as hostess/waitress. Dad would pick me up from my night shift at 2 a.m.

in his red VW Rabbit. He never complained about getting up in the cold night air for me. The car, which ran on diesel, had to be plugged in for easier starts in frigid temperatures. While I sprinted inside seconds after we pulled into the driveway, Dad would remain outside, orange extension cord in hand, plugging in the car while little icicles formed on his whiskers.

I'll always be especially thankful for that Bennigan's job, because it eventually led me to Bill. One afternoon, a regular customer asked if I was ever going to go to college. I had begun taking part-time classes, and working to earn enough to return to school. He told me about a job at the Chicago Board of Trade, where many of the companies paid for college and offered hours that would allow me to both work and attend classes. A few days later, I walked onto the trading floor. It was electric. People were shouting and waving their arms frantically. I made my way through the crowd and to a small desk right next to the 30-year-bond pit. My soon-to-be boss Tom asked, "Do you have a good set of lungs on you?"

"Definitely," I smiled.

"Can you run?"

"Absolutely, I was the fastest girl in sixth grade."

He and his partner laughed at me. "Well, Annette, you start Monday." I was clueless as to what the job entailed, but figured they would teach me. Most of it involved running. All day long I ran, grabbing papers and trading cards to bring them from one place to the next. The chaos there was strangely familiar…just like home, only minus the little ones. I loved it.

Bill

⁓

CHICAGO IS A GREAT CITY for falling in love. I met Bill in the early spring of 1993 at Four Farthings, a neighborhood bar. For me, it was not just love at first sight, but like retrieving something precious that you hadn't known you'd lost. While he talked, I found myself envisioning us through the years, growing old together, talking exactly as we were in that moment. When I spoke, he fixed his green eyes on me and listened intently to my every word. The conversation continued as we walked down Fullerton Avenue. I decided to share a scary truth, perhaps too early in our budding friendship. "Because I'm adopted, I just get this feeling I am all alone in the world." He seemed completely unfazed. "Really, you're adopted? Me, too." I felt that we were two kindred souls with a shared secret.

When we reached my apartment, he gave me a hug and left. I practically floated up the stairs, and grabbed the phone to call my sister Patti. "Guess what? I met the man I'm going to marry! I wanted you to be the first to know, and you can tell everyone on our wedding day!" She thought I was crazy, but said, "I'll make a note of it." Bill is the first person, besides my Dad, who made me feel like I was home.

We started dating. Bill worked the market's European shift starting his work day in the middle of the night and coming home at midmorning. My job took me from the Board of Trade to the Mercantile Exchange, which meant I was home by 3 o'clock. By 4, I was waking him up to do something fun—take a walk, have beers at Otis Bar, eat chicken wings at Yakzies, or watch football at Gamekeepers, which served the world's best Bloody Marys. He would be exhausted, but always rallied. Sometimes, Bill would have to head straight to work from our evenings out, but you can function on very little sleep when you are falling in love.

Bill's thing is sports—back then, he could spend hours immersed in football, baseball, hockey. There's never a break from sports when you are with a former college football player. My preference has always been the arts: music, movies, paintings, and literature. While we were (and are) both captivated by completely different interests, Bill was game to try anything (one of the things I find so endearing about him). He was willing to attend an opera or spend the afternoon at the Art Institute, so long as we were together. And it did not seem to bother him that whenever we went to the movies, I always chose romantic comedies. He did manage to fall asleep during a performance of Beethoven's Symphony No. 7 by the Chicago Symphony Orchestra—totally unforgivable! I smiled and gave him the slightest nudge. Embarrassed he looked at me, and said, "No Annette, I love it. I do!" I appreciated the sincere effort he made to participate in the things I love.

Bill was the first boyfriend who didn't want to change anything about me. He tolerated my silliness. It didn't annoy him that I ran more slowly than him, talked too much, or woke him up just after he'd fallen asleep. He even adored my fashion missteps—the sweats, leggings, oversized t-shirts…even my pea-colored, thrift-shop trench coat with the big green buttons. (The one I was wearing when we met!) All were a part of my cuteness, according to him. It has been years since I've worn it, but I could never give up that old coat—it is like a cherished picture that holds the memory of a day that altered all of my future days.

A few months into our relationship, Bill was transferred from Chicago to Bermuda. He promised he wouldn't go, that he couldn't leave me, but he didn't have much say in the matter if he expected to keep his job. I was angry and refused to speak to him when he called. He flew home only months later and, on a cold February day we trudged through the snow on the shore of Lake Michigan. "Where are we going? What are we doing in the snow?" I asked. We sat down together on an ice-cold bench, he handed me a box and whispered, "Will you marry me?" "Yes!" I said, with tears in my eyes. An hour later, he had to catch a flight back to Bermuda. We made our plans via phone, and I would join him in a month. My family threw a party for me in a bar close to where we grew up. My sister came out with a large sheet cake that read "Bon Voyage." I was off on my first adventure.

When I called home after meeting Bill, Dad could hear in my voice that I was in love. He and Mom (ever his loyal companion) drove the five hours from where they'd retired in Wisconsin to Chicago, where Bill planned to ask Dad for permission to marry me. The day we chose to meet dumped nearly twelve inches of snow on Chicago, but my parents traveled through blizzard conditions undeterred, even after one of their windshield wipers blew off along the way. At the end of our time together, Bill had not asked Dad for my hand. Dad, sensing that Bill might be nervous, said to him, "Bill, just in case you had anything to ask me, the answer is YES," and with that he gave him a wink. Bill shook his hand. I sensed my parents' overwhelming happiness for me. After they left, I thought about all the trips Dad made to get me from work and marveled that he still made those valiant gestures on my behalf.

Bill and I lived in Bermuda the entire year we were engaged, and it was one of the happiest times of my life. Bermuda brought color to my world, and with it, an endless array of blooming flowers. It was like something I'd seen in one of Mom's old *National Geographic* magazines—the kind of place you read or dream about. And now I was there, with my own true love. Even the moon appeared more luminous each night than it had the night before. It was delirious and enchanting. Even better than my dreams.

We spent our weekends on a pink-sand beach where I dreamt about and planned our wedding day. It was not the dress that

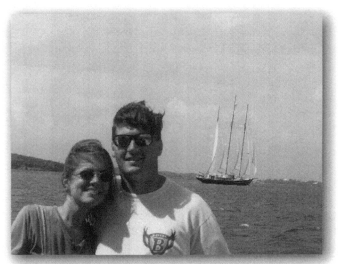

With Bill in Bermuda.

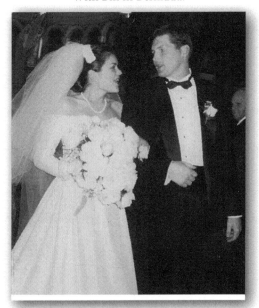

Our wedding day.

made this bride feel like a princess, it was my groom. We chose "Moon River" as our wedding song, from the movie *Breakfast at Tiffany's*. My favorite line from the film is when Audrey Hepburn says, "Nothing very bad could happen to you there." Being with Bill made me believe that nothing bad would ever happen.

Bill eventually grew antsy in Bermuda, and wanted to start our life back home. There was nothing I didn't like about life in Bermuda, but if he wanted to go, I was happy, as long as we were together. We were married at Chicago's St. Clement Church on April 22, 1995. As I held Dad's arm and turned to walk toward Bill, I felt all the joy that existed in the world was inside of me. I nearly burst with happiness. Bill smiled at me, and with each slow step toward him, I believed that all of my dreams had already come true.

The ceremony was very important to me; the reception, very important to Bill. Father Frank, the priest who oversaw our marriage preparation in Bermuda, flew to Chicago to preside over our ceremony. He delivered a homily that proved almost prophetic. He'd composed his remarks on the very turbulent flight, which he used as an analogy for marriage. "When a pilot is unable to see through thick storm clouds, he must rely on his instrumentation to land the plane. That is what your marriage should be like. You will not be able to see God, but trust in Him even when you cannot see through the storm." I don't remember every detail of our wedding day, but the priest's words endured, and they have haunted me.

The Fairy Tale

⁓

OUR FIRST HOME AS HUSBAND and wife was a tiny, extremely charming apartment on the third floor of a brownstone in Lincoln Park, with wooden floors, built-in bookshelves, and a fireplace. Bill was building his new company, and I was working at the Northwestern Memorial Hospital Foundation, and continuing my studies toward a Liberal Arts degree with a concentration in theology. Every class fascinated me, and I became a fearless participant in round-table discussions. I found a new appreciation for learning as I got older, no longer viewing it as work but as an absolute joy. The second summer we were married, I signed up for a course on the poet Dante; the bonus being that the class would be taught in Italy. Bill's company was doing well enough that he felt he could join me, so off we went. After one night in the dormitory in Rome, he and I ran off to a hotel very near to the Spanish Steps and opted to skip the academic portion of the trip. In exchange for lost credits, we took a month-long tour of one of the most romantic places in the world. It was a spontaneous decision, and there is not one thing I would change about it.

Each new morning, we awoke to coffee and set a plan for what we'd like to see. After days of quiet reverence spent viewing Madonnas and frescoes in churches and museums, Bill reached his saturation point, so we spent a day hiking through the Forum to view a different aspect of Rome's glory days. He may even have imagined himself a gladiator. We moved on to Venice. One starlit night, while strolling through Piazza San Marco, we saw a flyer for a concert and decided to attend. To my delight, the violin trio played my favorite Bach Concerto. Bill stayed awake and appeared as riveted as I was. We drove down the coast to Sorrento and visited Capri. The days dwindled, as we basked in the warm ocean breezes and played card games on the patio. We'd tasted our first Bellinis and enjoyed many a late-night Limoncello. As we looked out on the ocean, we knew it was time to head home. We didn't fill our bags with souvenirs from our Italian holiday, but we took with us treasures of another kind—beautiful memories.

Returning to a frigid Chicago, we weighed the benefits of our sophisticated, cosmopolitan city—with its fabulous food, charming neighborhoods, and small-town feel—with thoughts of purchasing a home of our own and starting a family. Bill asked if I would consider a move to his hometown, New Canaan, Connecticut.

I was torn, and so consulted my Dad. He didn't hesitate. "Go! If you follow Bill, you'll always be happy." That was unexpected. Did he want me to leave? Wouldn't they miss me? But, my father was my trusted advisor, and so we left Chicago. My time there with Bill remains untouched by anything sorrowful.

Connecticut

~~~

LIFE WAS FULL OF CHANGE. Dad always told me that change is the one thing you can count on. "It's inevitable," he promised. "Nothing else is guaranteed." As a child, it didn't scare me to think of change. In fact, I'd assumed that change was always good. (The simple innocence of youth!) I wished on many a nighttime star that someday I would find true love and live happily ever after; and now my wish had come true. Change meant only that more exciting things were about to happen. My world was beautiful, and it was there that I wanted to stop time.

We moved to the town where Bill grew up. It's not hard to understand why he wanted us to raise our family there. If there's such a thing as a perfect town, New Canaan may have been it. Being moved by beauty, I fell instantly in love with the landscape of our corner of Connecticut, with its winding roads lined with massive trees and rock walls. Each time he talked about his childhood, Bill lit up like a firefly. And he'd probably caught more than his fair share (of fireflies, I mean). He was a boy who loved to play. He'd spent countless hours playing stickball; rafting on the river with his best friend, Dave; and running through open fields with his dog, Schlitz. He captained his school's football team and seemed to have been a friend to all. I secretly wished I'd known him then, that boy of the '70s, in his cool plaid pants. Yes, this town would be the place—our place—and his idyllic childhood would carry on into the lives of our one-day children.

First Home, First Baby

~⁓

WHEN WE FIRST ARRIVED IN New Canaan, in the summer of 1997, we lived for a time with Bill's parents, John and Ellen. They were practical and pragmatic, highly intelligent, and ethical people whose moral code was built upon their own experience, trial and error, and inner voices. I suspect I made them just a little crazy with my neuroses, but they accommodated me. When we'd left Chicago, I'd still been working on my undergraduate degree; it was my mission to complete what I had begun. Before we left, I applied to and was accepted at Sarah Lawrence College. It was there I would proudly earn my bachelor's degree. At one crucial point when things got tough and the work load overwhelmed me, John said, "You'll always regret not finishing. Just do it!" Suddenly, I felt myself wanting Bill's parents to see me as someone who had what it took to persevere. I finished the long paper I put off on Canada's health care system. And I was grateful for John's wise counsel.

Bill's mom and I were similar in how passionately we clung to our ideas. But it was the topics over which we got fired up that often put us in opposition. At first, I thought my Catholic upbringing was the reason. Ellen had left the Church in early adulthood and could not grasp how any intelligent, thinking person could believe in God. I did not understand how any loving person could not. We were four very different people living under one roof, and common ground was hard to come by. There's one thing, though, on which his parents and I have always agreed—Bill has a beautiful heart.

Bill's Mom had delighted in him since he was a baby. His accomplishments made her proud. She wore his picture on her coat to every football game. She even made homemade birthday cards for him. For his eighth birthday, she wrote a poem, "It's Great to Be Eight." The few times that Bill found himself in trouble as a youngster, his parents defended him fiercely. He and his sister Bonnie were both adopted as babies. Bonnie, who is four years younger, was born in Boston and Bill in L.A. Bill was Bonnie's go to babysitter on the weekends. Instead of being his partner in crime while Mom and Dad were out, Bill made sure his parents believed Bonnie committed the crime. Usually, right upon their entrance home Bill was saying loudly, "Bonnie, you can't do that — Mom and Dad will see you!" Bill became an expert at tormenting his little sister, from chasing her with sticks, pelting her with snowballs, and tackling her during knee football. He says he did it all with love. Lucky for him she was a pretty good sport.

Because Bill was just a baby when his parents left California, his first and fondest memory of home was the yellow house on Mariomi Road. Most of his time was spent playing sports or playing with friends. The saddest event of his childhood was when his best friend Dave moved to Massachusetts. The Petersons were his second family. They lived just over the river and through the woods...seriously. He always felt welcome in their home, and they treated him as one of their own. In the winters they invited him to ski; in the summer it was crabbing and riding the ocean waves of Virginia Beach. Whatever the adventure, Bill was included. Mr. Peterson was so fond of Bill that he spoke at our rehearsal dinner, saying that he could not have loved him anymore if he was his own son.

I had never met anyone who reminisced about their childhood more than Bill. His parents did something right. They raised two very unique and special people. And yet, we had experiences with them where they seemed to impose what one might call "practical limits" on their love. (My own Dad had taught me that love knows no bounds. I know that, had we faced starvation, he would have given me his last morsel of bread. Bill's parents would have cautioned that such an act would ultimately save neither party.) Almost from the very start of our marriage, Bill's mom and dad thought our decisions together were outlandish, irresponsible, and sometimes just plain stupid. They said our dream house was a bastardization of a barn; it was not meant to be mean, but because they simply did not understand. Our love was big and it allowed us to believe that anything was possible.

It was also during our stay with the Rosses I found out I was pregnant. The newness of our circumstances coupled with my first pregnancy was almost too much for me. I felt anxious being so far from home, and was also plagued with concerns about what kind of mother I would be. Having grown up in a house overflowing with kids, I associated children with unrelenting chaos. When the trees started to change color in my first autumn in New England, excitement over life with Bill was mixed with a strange melancholy. I remember driving up route 124 and looking at the most vibrant colors I have ever seen—life and death merged as one. A new life was inside of mine and, while I rejoiced at what I understood to be the fruition of married life, I felt a loss. What would our life be like now that we were three? It was not sharing Bill; he had so much love to give. It was as it is so often with me, fear of the unknown.

Once we moved into our own house, a hundred-year-old Colonial with green shutters that was quintessentially New England, things went relatively smoothly. Despite my more reflective moments, we were in "the flow of life." Sarah Lawrence wanted a full two years of work in order to attain my bachelor's degree. I found the classroom setup there to be perfect—small classes, accessible teachers, and in-depth discussions. Because religion had always interested me, I took courses on the New Testament. I was captivated by my theology professor's profound understanding of the Bible, which gave me a different context in which to think about my favorite book. It was the word of God, but more than that. Professor Afzal taught us what he knew about who wrote it and when, and what life was like for the early Christians. They were people who had real struggles with their faith, something I could relate to. The days of me pulling one passage out for inspiration grew into something much richer. Professor Afzal humanized the text for us. (He even found connections to the lyrics of Bob Dylan, which he kept posted on his office door.) Sarah Lawrence, Professor Afzal, and Frank Roosevelt (my faculty adviser) all changed the course of my academic career. When I started there, my goal had been to complete a college degree. But, as I aspired for more, I remembered my Dad championing me to my mom ten years earlier, "Let her go, Betty." He'd been right.

For the first thirty years of my life, I'd always had easier relationships with males than with females, so I'd naturally envisioned that our baby would be a boy. The ultrasound said otherwise. "Can you check again?" I asked the technician. Having growing up with seven brothers, I was fairly confident that I could handle a son. I was nervous enough about becoming a mother, but had no idea how I'd respond to a daughter. When I told Dad we were expecting a girl, he said, "God gives you what you need, not what you want." His very words hung in the air. There was no doubt that he was right. Those special mother-daughter moments that never happened between Mom and me might now have a chance to be fulfilled with our little girl. It was up to me to build that bridge, which had never even existed with Mom. So, I was starting from scratch.

Natalie was born on a hot day in late March, 1998. Everything went very well. She was named after my childhood idol, Natalie Wood. Our Nat was the most beautiful baby I have ever seen. Every mom says that, but it was true. The moment the nurse put this little being in my arms I saw only *HER*, not her face, but her soul. The fullness of the moment swept me away. It was pure love. Even if we didn't know what we were doing, that first year of Natalie's life was so good. She didn't sleep, and taking her anywhere away from home was a recipe for disaster, but we did it anyhow. Hoping to nurse for a year, I learned how to maintain my milk production, and to make baby food from scratch. Nat and I attended music classes, and Gymboree gymnastics. It was tiring, but sublime. And, a part of me recognized that those sweet times with Natalie should be savored.

At the time of her birth, I was hard at work on my thesis about C.S. Lewis's *The Chronicles of Narnia*, a fairy tale with religious themes. Above Natalie's crib, I had a mural painted of the book's powerful Christ-like figure, the lion Aslan. What could be more perfect? It comforted me to think of her sleeping there. My professor Dr. Afzal had suggested that, as a devoted fan of C.S. Lewis and an expectant mother, I might enjoy analyzing the Narnia series. The seven books were quite unlike anything else I had read by Lewis. Fantasy fiction is not my preferred genre, but I enjoyed studying them. My favorite was *The Lion the Witch and the Wardrobe*—not because it was the most popular or because the Christian themes were more obvious, but because of the wardrobe. I was intrigued by the idea of a wooden cupboard containing the passage between two worlds, and by Lewis's mixing of magic and God. I received very good grades in all of my classes at Sarah Lawrence, and natural curiosity carried me all the way to graduation day, where I stood on the podium with a big smile, clutching my diploma in one hand and waving to Bill with the other.

I've yet to read the Narnia series with any of the girls. They remind me too much of where I thought I was headed as I first read them, and mark a time that is still difficult to look back on. (When I'd wanted to study the struggles of Saint Paul, my professor asked me, "Do you think you have ever suffered?" I responded with no hesitation, "Oh, yes," as I thought back on those periods of anxiety and subsequent emptiness that had sometimes enveloped me. Wasn't that suffering enough?) Back then, I was so certain of my beliefs that, if I ever encountered something that contradicted them, I could immediately counter them with what I knew to be "right." It was only real suffering that turned the sureness of my faith into shades of doubt.

Bill was doing well trading. When a beautiful property nearby came on the market, he said, "Come take a look at it with me." It was stunning. And expensive. We agreed that it was special and worth the risk. "Annette, worst case scenario it will be a great investment. Let's do it." Just days before it was officially ours, we stood in the front yard and I told Bill, "We're going

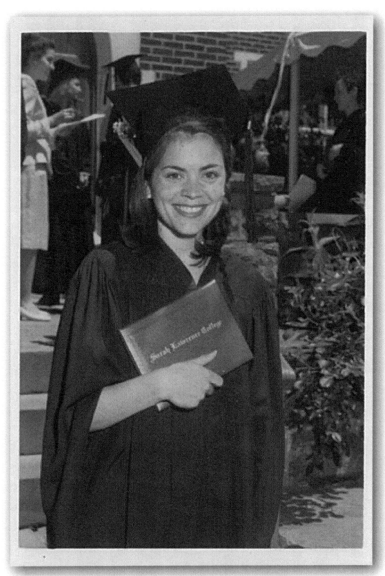

Graduating from Sarah Lawrence (1999)

to have another baby!" It was May of 1999, and we could smell the lilac trees.

The house on Hemlock Hill had once been part of a working farm and was made up of several small structures that, over time, had been joined by architects to create a wonderful, rambling old farmhouse. Old stone walls and a split-rail fence surrounded the property, which included a grove of tall white pines, large evergreens, pear, apple, and birch trees, a perfectly shaped maple, and two lovely lilac trees side by side. Along the street, we put in cherry trees, eventually planting one for each of our babies. The place was paradise for anyone who enjoyed flowers. There were bleeding hearts in the courtyard, rows of daffodils along the stone wall, lush hydrangeas, peonies, roses, butterfly bushes and Dad's favorite, a large bush of viburnum. The very first time he walked the property with me he said, "Annette, would you look at this!" He pinched off a bloom of tiny white flowers and handed it to me. "It smells like heaven," I said. From early spring to autumn the land was in a constant state of bloom. The final hurrah each year was provided by the pear trees, which held onto their dark auburn leaves long after the other autumnal colors had faded.

While not precisely enchanted (as much as I wished it had been), the grove of white pine trees along the side of our home was so prominent that, early on, we decided to name our home after them. "The Pines" was never made official, no plaque was ever engraved, but we joked about it to one other. "Let's go home," Bill would say. "The Pines await us."

The house was as distinct inside as it was out. The entrance was an unusually wide hallway, having once accommodated a row of animal stalls. The hall opened up into a large living room that looked out onto an expansive yard. The floors were a warm, wide-planked cherry wood; the winding staircase large enough for the girls to take their mattresses and slide down as though it were a sledding hill. During its renovation, the farm's silo had been converted into a wine cellar with a nursery above it. There were two stone fireplaces. We kept a fire going nearly every day in the winter. The first time we went to the house together, we drove up to the back entrance and rang the doorbell. A very kind woman opened the door, and my first thought was that we'd entered our own Narnia, a new land full of possibility and wonder.

My mom was quoted once in the local paper back home as saying that three meals a day and a roof over one's head were all that a child needed. To me, while food, shelter, and clothing are essential, they do not constitute "a home." The house I grew up in was not impoverished due to a lack of funds. It was lacking because Mom insisted that the curtains be drawn all day, even when the sunshine would have warmed a room. One can convince oneself that, by offering a hungry person crumbs, you're feeding them but, in truth, they remain malnourished. Starvation is as much an emotional condition as a physical one. I told myself that I would do things differently once I had a home and family of my own. During our years at The Pines,

I learned that love manifests in the little things—bedtime stories, glow-in-the-dark stars on the ceiling, patchwork quilts, and birthday parties. And yet I held onto a fear that I would continue the same cycle of emotional poverty I'd experienced growing up with my own children.

I couldn't have anticipated the transformation that occurred in her, but when my Mom became a grandmother, she became a gentler person. So sweet, especially with babies. I overheard a conversation she once had while playing with a very young Anna. Mom held a little plastic doll and, as she dressed it, explained each detail to Anna. "Now we're putting the sweater on the baby. Next we'll find the baby's socks and shoes..." Infancy was the stage of life my Mom related to best. She could have stayed there for hours, content with Anna and the dolls. This was her comfort zone, and I came to realize, her expertise.

Mom and Dad moved East in 1999. The timing was almost spooky, as if they foresaw that they would be needed. On an earlier visit to Connecticut, Dad had suffered a heart attack, and we'd found an excellent cardiologist whose care saved his life. Bill and I urged them to move closer to us, and they quickly agreed. Having them nearby made Connecticut feel more like my home, and I was enthusiastic about caring for them in their later years. In June, only a month after we moved into The Pines, Bill and I took a vacation (on what turned out to be our last trip sans wheelchair). Natalie stayed back with Mom and

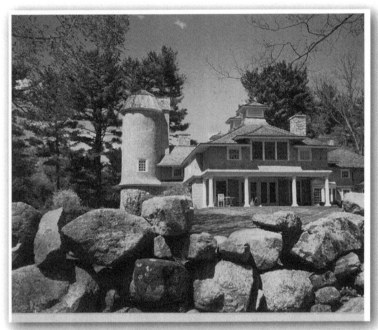

Our home The Pines.

Dad. It was the first time we were ever away from her. When we left, Nat who was almost 15 months old was not quite walking. Upon our arrival we opened the door, and she did a little run to greet us, arms wide open. Yes, Bill and Betty still had the knack. They looked so proud. Less than a year later, they were caring for us instead.

We had only lived at the farmhouse for six months when I was hurt, but it was home, and I longed to return there after my hospitalization. The day I transitioned from the rehab facility, the pine trees looked almost as sad as I felt. Being reunited with them eased my burden. They seemed to call to me and I answered back, in a whisper, "Hello, trees." Finally, I was home. Much later, Bill told me that he went outside that very same night, stood on the porch, and surveyed the trees. He asked them, "What just happened?"

The first time I entered the house in my wheelchair, everything felt dark and eerily quiet. My cherished white bulldog, Bella, greeted us at the door but swiftly ran away, bewildered at sight of this big clamoring device. "Hey, it's okay, Bella. We're home," I tried to reassure her.

Being home meant being a wife and a mother, *not* a disabled woman. Reluctant as I was to use it, a wheelchair wasn't out of

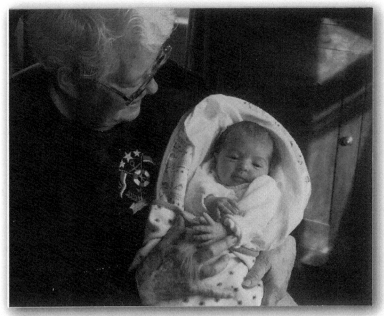

Mom with baby Natalie.

place within the confines of the hospital and rehab—places where people are sick, get better, and go home. But now this *thing* was to be a permanent fixture in our home. Was this the new me?

Grief

~

GRIEF TAKES HOLD FOR AS long as it will. There are stages one must pass through, and even when you think you've moved beyond one, it comes back again, only less intensely than before. At least, that's how it was for me. Elizabeth Kubler Ross wrote about the five stages of grief in her book, *On Death and Dying*. I was going to live, but the stages still applied, because a part of me *had* died. You don't have to lose your life to die.

Our friend Deacon John from Saint Aloysius Church in New Canaan waited for us in Bill's home office the day we came home. He had baptized Natalie and was close to our family. A man of deep faith, he listened as I went to battle with the forces within. I was hopeful. I was despairing. I wanted to be home, but wanted to leave. I was a mother and a wife. I kept thinking that I wanted to do what was right, but I didn't know what that was anymore. I longed to know what God wanted me to do. Where was He? If there was one answer I wanted from the Deacon, it was an explanation for why God had chosen the day of Anna's birth to take a holiday. Where was God when the chemicals choked the nerves in my spine? Isn't He always with us? He missed His part, and what happened would affect not only me, but also Bill, Natalie, and Anna. "John," I begged him, "why did this happen? Can you offer any insight? Did I do something to bring this about?" It wasn't even two months since the night of my injury, but I had already asked the same questions ad nauseam. Sometimes, the only solace one can offer is to be with someone in their sorrow, and Deacon John sat with us as we cried and tried to make sense of the unpredictability of life.

On his way out that day, Deacon John said, "Annette, this just came to me. You need to let Bill guide you. He will bring you through this."

"But how?" I asked him. "His faith is not as strong as mine."

"I just know that if you follow his lead, things will be all right." His words reminded me of what my Dad had said when I asked him whether or not we should move to New Canaan. "Follow Bill and you will always be happy."

There was nothing else to do. "Of course, John," I responded. "I will do that. I will try."

Deacon John was right. I would need to rely heavily on Bill. I wasn't ready to do anything else. There was no way I could run the house, take care of the girls, and organize a therapy schedule on my own. Being inside our home with Bill and the girls was the only place I felt safe. Had I decided to draw the curtains, I would have officially become a recluse like my mother. But I resisted closing off entirely. But, for a time, Bill became *the* person from whom I derived all of my happiness. The other aspects of life were too difficult and burdensome—mothering, therapy, even the once simple act of showering. When the water hit my legs, it felt like the pellets from a BB gun were blasting them. The pain wasn't real—at least not on the surface—but caused my nerve endings to burn intensely. And it made something I used to enjoy an experience to endure.

We had extra hands at home, but Bill could sense when I needed something to be done by *him* and no one else. We'd hired Helen, an attentive night nurse, to help with Anna. Bill's parents and mine were not at an age where they could be up all night with a newborn. And Bill needed his sleep, too. Most nights, though, I couldn't sleep and stayed up late watching old movies. If I was able to close my eyes long enough to dream, I always saw myself walking. But usually, I was awake, reading the captions on the television so as not to wake Bill, and listening to the sounds of the night. A family of raccoons ran back and forth from the knot in our tree to the garbage at the side of the house. Their long claws scratched the driveway as they scurried along. Perched on the branches anxiously waiting for dinner were their children, I think I counted at least three. It delighted me to think our garbage provided their nightly feast. But the sound I most looked forward to was the owls. I usually heard them right before the first light of morning. Their song was lonely, and at the same time, comforting. I came to know in a profound way what it meant to be a "night owl." Whenever I heard Anna's cries from down the hallway, I couldn't bear the thought of a stranger comforting her. If she woke Bill and he noticed the look on my face, he'd ask, "Annette, do you want me to get her?" I knew he was exhausted but would nod "yes," anyway. I needed to feel a mother's closeness with her. But the reality of the situation was such that, if Anna needed to be walked back to sleep, Bill was doing the walking, not me. And he did. This became our routine. The nurse felt badly about standing idly by, but it was what I needed, and Bill understood in a way that others could not.

Anna was such an easy baby that Bill did get an occasional night's rest, but he was deeply involved in all my other care as well; helping with my therapy and learning how to stretch my contracted legs. He was attuned to my muscle spasms, and knew how not to push against what my body resisted. Once, an over-zealous therapist pulled my Achilles tendon with such force, my heel bone fractured. Bill never once caused me an injury or additional pain. If I couldn't sleep, he tried to stay up with me until I was finally able to rest. But, it was the *emotional* burden that he shouldered that helped the most. I could share with him how I honestly felt, and he never judged. I exposed feelings that were not what I wanted my husband of only five years to know. If I hated everything about a day, he promised that tomorrow would be better. I never had to sell him on the idea that I was still me. He believed it before I did.

In the hospital, he would climb into my hospital bed with me instead of staying on the couch. The bed was small, and crowded (often I was holding Anna), and people were coming in and out of the room, but I think he wanted me to know that he was not afraid of me; that no matter what, he was not going to let me go.

At home we tried to resume the same level of intimacy we had always shared, but it didn't go well at first. Things were not the same; they did not feel the same. My body felt like it did not belong to me. Because Bill is an open, sensitive, and loving person, he never made these early attempts stressful. And, he never showed concern for himself. I felt like a colossal failure and was angry that something so beautiful was taken away from us. Bill was patient; he did not share my gloom and doom. (He *did* think it would help if I could stop crying every time we tried to have sex.)

"This isn't working for me," I confided in my doctor, who was not only an excellent physiatrist, but a wonderful friend. "Annette," she said gently but firmly, "get out of your head. Bill is not judging you." It was true. If my unpredictable bodily functions bothered or repulsed him, he was too kind to say it. He was only full of acceptance, love, and a sense of humor. So often, I wondered if I would have felt the same had our roles been reversed. I wanted us to be as close as we had always been, and so I needed to approach my body with curiosity, to learn about it; and for me, that was brave.

It was an act of discipline not to think about how much my body had changed. My skinny, atrophied legs were a distraction. When I saw them unclothed, I immediately felt sad. There was the additional problem of my bladder, which responded to every move we made with an urgent message to race to the bathroom. With little warning, I'd cry out, "Bill, I have to go...NOW!" He'd jump up, grabbing me like a football, headed for the end zone. If we didn't make there within seconds, it was too late. In the beginning, the situation was too raw for me to laugh about, but eventually we had to.

Bill and I kept trying and, slowly, I started to accept that "different" did not always equal bad. Eventually, we discovered something new and, surprisingly, it brought us even closer. If only walking were that easy. In marriage, sexual intimacy is not merely physical, but a coming together of two souls; it is a union that is sacred. I had always believed this, and allowed it to come to fruition in our married life. My vulnerable self was safe with Bill. With the disability came a test of sorts, and we passed. Nothing was altered in a way that could be considered diminished, and everything I hoped to believe about such a union was realized. People are often curious about the sex lives of the disabled, and some feel no shame in probing for specifics. I've certainly been asked. The answer is intensely private. But we do have five daughters, so I think we figured it out.

Alison

MY NEXT DOOR NEIGHBOR MORLEY came to visit only days after we were home. As we sat together in the living room, I stared out the double pane windows onto the lawn. It was late February and everything appeared dead. She noticed the blank look in my eyes and said, "Annette, I think you should consider getting some help, not just to help you walk, but to help you adjust to what has happened." Both the hospital and rehab center had provided psychological assistance, but she was right, it hadn't been enough. She gave me the name of a woman in town.

Alison came so highly recommended that I was hopeful. "Therapy is hard work." she said. And that was true. You must be ready to engage honestly, confront your deepest feelings, and reveal your innermost fears. (I'd sought therapy before, for my anxiety, even seeing a specialist in panic disorder. But I now needed something more comprehensive.) Some days you don't want to do the work, but you do it anyway, and that is when the magic happens.

"I'm scared about my relationship with Anna," I told Alison. "Will I somehow hold my injury against her, not intentionally, but because this happened the day she was born? How will I separate the painful outcome from the gift of her life? Am I bad mother?"

"You *will* love her, Annette, as much as you love Natalie, and you'll have an even more special relationship with her for having gone through this." I didn't know if that was possible, but if she believed it, I would trust her.

It didn't feel intimidating to be vulnerable with Alison. When I shared with her the mishaps that Bill and I had as we worked toward a healthy sex life, or of the many times I had an accident before reaching the bathroom, she never once flinched. She was a master at unpacking the issue to uncover what was at its core. Not having control of my bladder repulsed me. I could not fathom that it was actually me. It took such a long time to be able to roll my eyes about it and say, "It's no big deal," and mean it.

The cottage Alison worked from did not have a bathroom, so she became familiar with the urgency of this issue. When I really had to go, there was no stopping me. Once, we made use of the only thing available—a large wooden bowl. "You'll want to throw this away now," I said, sheepishly. She laughed. I felt super embarrassed, but she was unflappable. The loving way she handled things turned these awkward moments into lasting memories.

Alison doted on me during our time together, becoming almost a surrogate mother. If my lower back hurt, she had a bag of beads for me to lean against. Her couch was infinitely cozier than my wheelchair, so once I transferred, she would quickly adjust my feet on the ottoman. If they were throbbing and burning from the neuropathy I experienced so often, she would hold my feet in her hands until the sensation calmed. Once she knew she had addressed any of my immediate physical needs, we would begin.

Alison said that, often, I already knew the answers, but that it was her job to bring them to a more conscious place. Whether I hated myself, or God, this was the place where I could say it out loud. Scream it, if necessary. She provided the room for me to be small. I was not ready to be anything else. Her objective was not to change my point of view. If I found disability repugnant, that was fine, she validated exactly where I was in that moment. Then, in a subtle but brilliant move, she would propose a different perspective; a new possibility. The world was bigger, the mystery greater, and the hope not as elusive as I'd thought. She instinctively knew when I could handle her pearls of wisdom. I would ask, "When will it get better? When will the sadness dissipate?" She would look at me intently. "It will always be with you, but you can make it into something beautiful. From this experience you will find wisdom, more strength than you ever knew you had, and a purpose," she promised. She called it my "hero's journey."

My time with Alison was a respite from a life in which I felt constant guilt for my feelings. People were being incredible, helpful, and patient. And although grateful to them, I remained at war—not with the doctors, or lawyers, or even God—but with myself. Did I have a right to be upset? Had I only desired an easy life and felt anger when it was taken from me? That seemed so small. Although we were in complete privacy, I could not stop thinking that, if my Dad could hear what I was saying, he would be disappointed with me. Alison felt compassion for our family, not pity. And, I needed that. I wanted someone to say they were sorry for what had happened, and she did. She would look directly into my eyes and say, "Annette, I am so sorry." The words lightened the load. I'm not even sure why. Sometimes I needed her to cry with me, and she did. A good cry often gave me the strength to face one more day. I had been so close to my "happily ever after." I know I'm not the first, nor the last person to feel this way. Sometimes, when I'm on a plane, I look at the people around me and wonder about them. Are they happy? Do they feel just as disappointed in life as I do? What if they do? How does any one of us have the capacity to bear life's sorrows and uncertainty? I spoke to Alison about these thoughts, about the loss of my dream, and she explained that the loss was shared, a part of the collective loss we all feel. "Nothing happens in a vacuum, Annette."

After the initial shock of our loss (and many talks with both Alison and Deacon John), Bill and I were able to recreate something special at The Pines. It wasn't what I had once envisioned, but it was happy, and perhaps the biggest reason was Mary. We hired her after we no longer needed a night nurse. Anna was sleeping well with us, but we needed an extra pair of hands while I continued to work on strengthening my legs.

Mary quickly became a main cog in the wheel, and one of the best friends I have ever had. We discovered after hiring her that she shared a devotion to the Catholic faith, the Blessed Mother in particular. It almost seemed that she'd been handpicked by God for our family. She was someone I could talk to, pray the rosary with, and get advice from. Could anyone suit me more perfectly? I told her everything, and she cared for me as much as she did the girls. When I came back from a training session she was ready with a tuna melt. If she noticed I looked tired she offered to do an extra load of laundry or make the family dinner. She even cooked for Mom and Dad when they came over.

During the Mary years, our home ran like a finely tuned machine and, when she took time off, she replaced herself with someone just as competent, such was the extent of her commitment to our family. When Ingrid couldn't find her "lappy" (a favorite blanket), Mary was sure to find it. She knew where *everything* was. I was able to love, and hug, and squeeze my girls, and Mary made sure they were wearing socks and shoes. Her presence allowed me to place full attention on my legs.

Also because of Mary, we regained enough energy to extend beyond ourselves and resurrect our once-social life. So, we entertained. Each year we hosted a party on the Saturday after Thanksgiving. My trainers attended, and our closest friends from the neighborhood. Some years, nearly 100 people were there. These were catered events and the girls dressed up for them. Days after the party we were still eating the leftovers, opening the hostess gifts, and talking about how we couldn't wait for next year. We felt very much a part of things then, people were involved in our life—and in my dream to walk—and we joined in celebrating their milestones with them. Life was full, the only missing ingredient was my ability to walk, and yet the love in our home was palpable. I never wanted it to end.

We all believed that it was only a matter of time before I walked again. Through rigorous physical therapy, I was able to command movement in my legs. They were not technically paralyzed, only dormant and receiving too weak a signal to function properly—something akin to a dim light bulb needing more wattage. The problem was in harnessing that additional wattage. I could move both of my legs, my right being just a bit stronger, but my left had less spasms so that made them equal in terms of functionality. With the help of AFO's (ankle foot orthotics) which were necessary to keep my feet from dragging and a walker, I could carefully walk. It did not require focus as much as it did stamina. Part of my therapy routine was to walk the driveway. Someone was needed to steady the walker and someone to push the chair behind me for when I needed rest. Slowly, very slowly, I would make my way down the path toward the street. Eventually, my endurance was such that I was able to walk the entire length of Hemlock Hill. There was weight through my legs, but a great deal of the effort was my upper body, and sheer will. The walk was exhausting, and also invigorating. I do not think I fully realized the toll it was taking on my shoulders, arms, and lower back to compensate for what my legs could not do, but I read that the motion of walking sometimes awakened the connections and so I continued to get up and do it every day. My entire body felt the strain at night. Every muscle fiber was at work trying to making up for the ones that were still sleeping. Each time I made the journey, people who were driving by waved, honked or stopped to wish me well. Their positive reinforcements helped me take one more step.

We outfitted a home gym, brought in therapists and trainers, and investigated every alternative modality in our efforts to create a plan for success. I felt guilty about the amount of time and resources involved but knew that, had this happened to one of the girls, or to Bill, we would leave no stone unturned.

We were told by numerous physicians and therapists that the odds were not with us. But we also knew that, should I achieve my dream, it would benefit us all. If sheer force of will was a significant part of the equation, I could see myself like the underdog, Rocky Balboa (my hero), running up all those steps, music blasting; and I would be victorious!

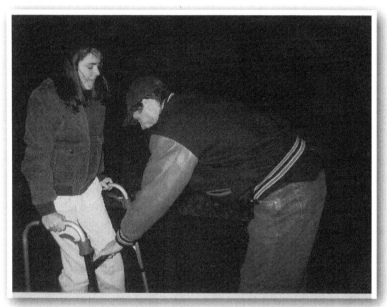

Rehabbing with Bill in the driveway. (2003)

The facility we went to after leaving Yale hadn't shared my "Rocky" vision. Therapists who work with spinal-cord-injury patients teach them how to live in a wheelchair, coaching them into accepting a new normal. But at that time, I was about ten years away from anything like accepting that I would not walk again. Once I'd proved to them that I would not be a burden to society (only to everyone in our home), they were happy to let me leave to pursue whatever treatments we wanted at our own expense. The mass of grey walls, floor mats, and short-tempered nurses who detested patient care made it that much easier to leave behind.

The one positive aspect to on-site rehab was the rapport and camaraderie one builds with other patients. The paths that bring each of us there are unique, and is a stunning reminder that life can change in an instant. One woman who, like me, was also in her early thirties, told me, "I'm here because my husband tried to kill me. He was cutting down a tree, called me outside to watch him, and told me where to stand. The tree fell on me, and knocked me over. He was smart, and knew which way it would fall." She was adamant that he purposefully positioned her in harm's way. "Couldn't you run the other way?" I asked in horror. "There was no time," she said.

Another frail, soft-spoken woman sat stiffly in her chair. A quadriplegic, she looked almost lifeless, yet she could manage a smile and her gentle voice was always kind. As she stared vacantly at the walls, you could sense her despair. Never too shy to ask a question, I asked her what had happened. "I slipped on a piece of lettuce at a restaurant on my way to the bathroom." I couldn't believe it. She couldn't either. But there she was.

"Who will take care for you when you go home?" I asked. Her parents were too old to become her caregivers and she had no one else to help. "I may have to stay in some kind of facility for a long time," she said, with no hint of emotion. The outcome of her lawsuit against the restaurant would likely not be determined for years. So many severe cases leave a person in the care of strangers who they can only hope will treat them with compassion. I realized that, as tough a break as I'd gotten, I was still very lucky.

I recalled an unsettling book I'd read in college, *All God's Mistakes*, about detecting genetic anomalies in unborn babies. Looking at myself and my fellow patients, I felt that *we* were God's mistakes or, more accurately, God's forgotten children. It didn't seem right that we should survive our injuries only to end up defective and abandoned. Even so, we shared a sort of gallows humor. One young man I saw frequently at rehab would inevitably respond to my greeting with, "Annette, I'm one more day above the dirt." Was that good or bad, I'd asked. "Not sure," he'd say. Ours was not a club you'd wish to join, but we became each other's allies among the medicine balls, ropes, and weight machines.

Opposition and Doubts

IT'S BEEN SAID THAT THERE are no atheists in foxholes. As disappointed as I was with God, my pleas to be saved did not cease. Prayer was the answer. There are 150 psalms in the Bible —essentially cries for help and safety. Had I written down my own, I could have added 150 more. Deacon John believed with all of his being that I should stay close to God, even in my state of nothingness. I explained that I prayed and even begged God for a miracle every day, all day, endlessly. "God won't leave me like this, right?" Quietly, John replied, "Annette, I honestly don't know."

My feelings about everything seemed to be in constant opposition, grateful for all of the good that was still in place—healthy children, a loving husband, a wonderful home—but agony, rage, and depression over my legs, and even more at not being able to control my tumultuous emotions. It was an endless cycle that not even sleep would alleviate. I began to envision my family's life without me, and contemplated swallowing a bottle of pills. (Could I actually ever take my own life? God forbid, but the thoughts were there.)

Bill might actually be better off. He'd easily find someone else—he was young, handsome, full of life. And there was his greatest attribute, his huge heart. Sure, it would be sad for the girls to never know me, but growing up with me as their mom would affect their lives in ways I could never predict or control. It didn't seem fair to them. Maybe I questioned if love was really enough. Infants and toddlers need protection and security. Could I adequately provide that? I truly believed I might not be enough for them.

Early on, I had no idea how to cope with the barrage of insensitive remarks and judgmental opinions that came my way. Everyone seemed to have lost their filter. I overheard a friend tell her daughter that I had help at home because my daughters "needed two mommies" since I was in a wheelchair. It was assumed that I no longer desired the same things I once had, that my expectations had automatically diminished. But, why would they have? Friends, acquaintances, and even strangers felt competent to share what they believed my limitations should be. There was a growing consensus that I should not have a larger family, and they said as much. One friend who was actively trying to conceive said, "What gives you the right to have more children?" There was little I could say to that, so I quietly replied, "I'm really sorry you feel that way."

Good therapy taught me that people will project their "stuff" on you, and it's not personal. Eventually, I reached a point where very little that was said really penetrated. It wasn't that I was immune, but I understood (and truly believe) that such comments were more thoughtless than intentionally hurtful.

A day before attending a friend's party, the hostess called to ask a favor. "Annette, I know you're attached to your wheelchair, but it's going to be crowded in the house. Would you mind leaving it outside and having Bill carry you in?" The word I found most offensive was "attached," as if my wheelchair was my security blanket. I was not Linus from *Peanuts*. The chair was, like it or not, my mobility, my legs. We went to the party. Bill carried me inside, and dispensed me on a chair where I remained for the evening. My friend was an extremely bright, sophisticated woman, yet she lacked the sensitivity to understand how her request might make me feel. No one wanted to leave the wheelchair behind more than me.

Prayer was a daily part of my parents' life. Growing up, should anyone in our family ever need something—a job, a good grade, or to locate our missing pet rabbit—they would pray about it. Although it would prove to be a disadvantage later, from my earliest memories, I believed that God always answered my prayers exactly as I asked. He was with me, watching me—not in judgment, but delight. There was no separation between His world and mine. Perhaps that is a gift of childhood; to see all as one. God was my first real friend. I convinced myself that He had everything to do with how well (or how badly) a person's life went. There was no need to develop a more comprehensive construct; it was simple faith, the faith of a child. In my life with Bill, our little

Natalie, and Anna on the way, I had felt so blessed. To me, our good fortune meant that God's light was shining directly on us.

When things began to fall apart, that light went dark. Alison called this my "God in a box" theology and knew its black-and-white nature would always fail me. God was bigger than I was allowing Him to be. I have friends whose injuries are far worse than mine, and yet they feel blessed. Their authenticity startles me, and I see how much I've changed. God is there, whether you realize it or not. It may feel like he evades us when we stumble, but faith is not a feeling, it is not consolation. I do not think God gives it to us in advance, and then we have it like a pair of shoes. As each day unfolds, our faith has to be reestablished; at least it has gone that way for me.

To be sure there is a constant gnawing within that along the way I have lost my inherent goodness. The author Vladimir Nabokov suggested that suffering can make us callous. Am I as kind as I once was? Then I find a stray animal, and see every frail person in one lost creature. I hope suffering has made me embrace humanity and not recoil from it, but it shifts. We are not one thing and then remain that way. When I get up and climb down the stairs in the morning, I am fighting off the urge to stay in bed and give in. We never know when we reach our breaking point. My fight becomes an act of will, my every response in the day begs the question, "Will I give in?"

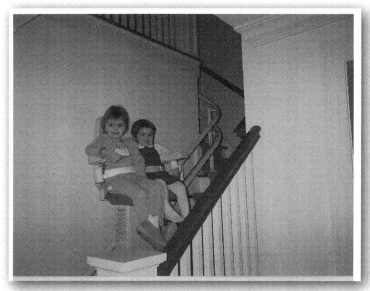

The stair climber at The Pines with Natalie and Anna

While I was in the hospital newly injured, people brought me many books on faith and suffering. My questions were turned from anesthesiologist to God. The books helped me to feel less alone, but didn't provide answers to the "why" questions: "Why me?" "Why was my life unfolding in this way?" Was it sin? Karma? Bad luck? Maybe if I had enough faith, if I really believed, I would walk again. The doctors had done what they could. Now it was God's turn. So began our odyssey to find every healing Mass in the Northeast.

We heard many stories of people liberated from crutches and wheelchairs, and witnessed the faithful fall to the floor when "slain in the spirit." I held out hope that I'd wheel into one of these churches and walk out, unaided. But nothing like that ever happened to us, and although I heard stories we never actually witnessed a miracle. Still, I craved the supernatural, the inexplicable; something that superseded the laws of the natural world. So we sought out individuals we'd heard were endowed with the gift of healing. It was one strange experience after another. With each new encounter, I tried to keep an open mind. One man came to the house with a group of people who stood in a circle and recited prayers together. He knelt in front of me and held my feet in his hands as he bowed his head. "Did you feel that?" he asked. "One of your legs lengthened. It was shorter, but now it's not." I'm not sure how he thought that would benefit me, and of course it hadn't. Strike one.

A woman who performed "magic" in the back woods of Connecticut claimed to have placed a steel rod into my leg to make it stronger. No surgical procedures had taken place that afternoon, but she was definitive. Strike two.

A friend heard about a woman with a weeping statue of the Blessed Virgin Mary. We entered a dimly lit room filled with religious icons. At the very center stood the statue, nearly identical to the one I prayed to the night of Anna's birth…the statue that has accompanied us on every move. I trust the Blessed Mother to watch over us, and there she stood, a statuette with tears trailing down the front of the blue-painted wooden gown. The homeowner was a humble, faithful woman, not seeking money or acclaim. She encouraged me to get out of my wheelchair and walk toward the statue. "If you just believe, she will help you. Try!" I didn't believe, but I tried. Strike three.

Eventually, we stopped looking for a mystical healer. Maybe these "miracles" are personal revelations only intended for those who have them. We stopped asking people to pray over me. In the book, *When Bad Things Happen to Good People*, the author concluded that God is good and loves us, but lacks omnipotence. I disagree. It's not that He's powerless, but that He doesn't work on command. It does not matter what you know, until you comprehend. No profound truths could penetrate the wall I'd built. Disappointed and disillusioned, I smiled on the outside but something was changing on the inside. A friend from Church took me to lunch. As we waited for our food she asked angrily, "What has happened to you, don't you know that Jesus is still hanging on the cross?" It did not matter. Nothing, not even God, was getting in. There was no room for Him.

The only person who was allowed in my spiritual tornado was Bill. He was not afraid of my deep sorrow, or my need to go to healing Masses. He knew me well enough to let me run this show, and trusted that eventually I would work through it. What kind of person does that for you? A husband should, but doesn't always. Not to say that each time he went along happily. Once, he threw my wheelchair across the driveway in protest. He was sick of it, tired of doctors, and appointments, and tired of people telling us why I was not being healed. They pointed the finger and made judgments, usually about something we were doing wrong. The idea that what happened was somehow our fault began to take hold, and once again I acted from a place of fear. I had the house blessed once and then again in hopes that any negative oppression would be released. This brought out the worst in me, and Bill, knowing on some level that this was what I needed, obliged—he never said no, but that is not to say he always agreed, hence the wheelchair slaying. God felt far away, but while He took some time off, Bill was with me in Hell.

After I'd been in my wheelchair for a year, I met a man who was a quadriplegic. Michael had no fine motor movement at all, which means he required a caregiver for even the most rudimentary functions. While I visited him in the hospital as he healed from an infected pressure sore, I found the courage to ask him,

"Why are you always at peace?" I sensed that he had experienced something special, even extraordinary.

He told me, "Right after I was injured, as I lay in my hospital bed filled with despair, I turned to look toward the window. Seated next to me was the Virgin Mary, dressed in a blue gown, her hands folded in prayer. I blinked, and she was gone."

"Were you dreaming?"

"No," he said. "I felt her presence, and I know now that this life is nothing."

And yet, the father of my friend had a very different experience. "I pray every night for Michael to get the use of his hands back," he said, "every single night, and I won't ever stop." His face looked pained. It was his boy, and he was hurt in a swimming accident when he was only 15. Now his boy was a man who could not tie his shoes. He and his wife cared for their son, and to witness their devotion from the outside was beautiful. To live it, I am sure, was something else entirely. The one encounter with Mary gave Michael peace, but that was not a gift he could give his father. The Saints say that suffering is a gift, but how much suffering is enough for God?

If you believe in God you seek His consolation. How we recognize it is intensely personal. God seemed to be talking to everyone except for me. So many times strangers stopped to tell me they had a feeling I would walk again. One lady in a bright pink dress chased the family down the street just to say, "Girl, when I passed you just then I had the strongest feeling that you would be healed, up and not just walking, but running!" She leaned over to hug me. When anyone said that it made me cry, it was exactly what I longed to have happen. Was it God? But, I had to stop asking Him for the miracle of walking or to make Himself known. To grow, I needed a new prayer. "Help me to find the grace to accept your will." That was it. It wasn't surrender; it was exhaustion. I had no fight left. People suffer; it's the human condition. Did I think I was exempt? I could not condemn myself for wanting to escape my fate. After a long break from healers and healing services, I went back to Mass, but with a different approach. God did not need to perform a miracle. Like Thomas, I longed to feel the wounds, to know for sure, but it started to become clear that my path would be one of finding Him in the abyss. I prayed that I would be strong enough not to succumb to despair again. Despair puts a veil over us. And, as for supernatural occurrences, I no longer sought them.

Looking Back
(Sometimes Fondly)

~

MANY PRIESTS HAVE SHARED WITH me that I should not be concerned with this life, but the afterlife. The here and now feels real to me, even if it is only a dress rehearsal for the perfection that awaits us. Without a miracle or cure I will live out the days without the use of my legs. A saint-like person would possess the faith to override their negative emotions about such a fate. Why couldn't I get in touch with my best self and do the same? Mother Teresa did her work with the poor receiving no consolation from God for years. And yet while in her presence, no one knew or felt her interior emptiness. Can we be who we are not?

One night we arrived home to find a cat waiting for us under our car. A can of tuna later, we had a new family member. Similar scenarios have led to our accumulation of dogs, rabbits, and injured birds as well. Anything that's left out in the vast expanse alone, I want to care for. Or maybe it is that abandoned child inside of me that still seeks a place to belong. There is an inherent goodness I want for everyone and everything. I do not feel this comes from my exterior self but the deep recesses of my soul. That gives me hope.

Not everyone with a disability feels confined. However, for me, it is true to say that I did. There were frustrations and complications from the onset. On my first day of outpatient therapy, a woman rolled up to greet me. She'd fallen off of a second-story porch while holding her six-week-old baby. Her newborn was unhurt, but she had broken her back and was left a paraplegic. "Are you on medication?" she asked. "Because you're going to *need* it, if you're going to consider raising a baby in a wheelchair." Within a year of her accident, her husband had divorced her, and she was left to care for her daughter on her own. I've since learned that many marriages don't survive a wife's sudden disability. Her story was completely sad, but I dismissed our depressing conversation. I planned to walk with my girls. Until then, I would adapt to mothering from a chair. But the shadow she cast seemed to loom over my efforts.

Every move I made with the girls in tow was awkward and bumbling. When Natalie was two she was capable enough to be quite helpful. Anna was an infant. I never felt in command when they were little, quite the opposite; I felt Natalie could do more for my safety than I could for hers. There was no place this more evident than at the park. Underneath the swing set the ground was carpeted in wood chips, which made my wheels spin like a tire stuck in the mud. Natalie patiently waited next to the swing as I navigated that obstacle. Then she waited a bit longer for me to find my place behind her. After fastening her comfortably into the swing, I would give her a quick push and quickly move into position to be able to duck as the swing returned. Eventually, we would find a rhythm that allowed me to push her and also protected my face from a collision. But then, as kids do, she'd want to try something else. She loved the slide, especially when I'd climb out of my chair, crawl up the slide, and set her on my lap. "Let's go!" I'd cry, and down we'd sail. My strength was pretty good, but my spastic bladder was sometimes overwhelmed by too many transfers in and out of the chair. Aside from the occasional "accident," I often collected splinters in my behind (that I didn't feel). And then there were the other moms who ran lightly, push swings without fear of being hit in the forehead, and climbed ladders; always keeping up with and holding tightly to their little ones. I would never again be that quick.

Fear hampered my longing to being free with my daughters. I needed to consider that my desire to interact with them could cost me an additional injury. It was too easy to get hurt. And

I was painfully aware how another setback would burden Bill. I continued to try, for a while, but my efforts to overcome my limitations just reinforced my brokenness. My small victories at the playground did not outweigh the feelings of inadequacy. In time, I decided it was best to stop going. The park, the pool, and the ice rink would be "things to do with Daddy." But nighttime was for me, Natalie and Anna. While Bill worked in his office, the girls crawled into bed with me. I made up an entire series of what we came to call the "Darcy Stories" about a little girl who wore a different colored ribbon in her hair each day. Darcy lived in our house and had many adventures there. Each time I finished, they begged for more. "Please, Mom! What else did Darcy do?" After story time I would sing them to sleep usually ending with the Beatles song, "I Will": "Love you forever and forever love you with all my heart, love you whenever we're together love you when we're apart." Once asleep, I lay awake and wondered what kind of mom I would have been, walking with two little toddlers by my side from morning 'til night. When thoughts like that tormented me, I had to have the self-discipline to turn them off. We still craved normalcy, and fought to achieve it. Family vacations were special—time away from the routine, from therapy, from stress. We sought to create new memories for the girls, and for us. In truth, though, it was much easier to stay home at The Pines.

Anna was always comfortable around new people. Sitting on the beach, Bill and I would watch her toddle off to make friends with families on blankets twenty yards away. "Do you think she'll come back?" we'd say to each other. It may have been her second-child nature, but we couldn't help thinking that she hadn't properly bonded with us. Natalie stayed close and seemed very much the loyal first-born child. She never once admitted to feeling embarrassed by me, but I suspect she did.

When Anna first started preschool, she spoke up, "Mom, kids ask me why you're in a wheelchair."

"And, what do you tell them?" I asked.

"I just say I don't know."

I asked her, "Do you feel weird having me at your school?"

She didn't answer readily, but eventually said, "Yes, Mom. I love you but I don't like that you're different and people look at you."

"Why do you care if people look at me, if I don't?" I was really angry. "If I'm okay with it, can't you be?"

Bill overheard the conversation and chimed in. "Anna, don't do this to your Mom. You're hurting her feelings!"

Although it was hard for Bill to see it then, he had a very difficult time bonding with Anna. He could not stop himself from making the connection between her and what happened to me. In some ways it was in defense of me. Had Natalie been the one to admit how it made her feel when kids stared at me, Bill would have understood. But because it came from Anna, it struck a nerve. But there was no doubt that he wanted her to be close to us, being close was the kind of family we were determined to be.

Literally from birth, Anna was used to many different people looking after her. While Bill attended to me, it was my parents, Bill's folks, my sister Patti, and my brother Bruce who cared for Anna. Helen helped us at night, and it was no surprise that Anna became attached to her. One night I lay in bed, my legs throbbing, and listened to her cries. She was my baby and I wanted to be the one to soothe her tears. I climbed into the chair and wheeled to her pretty pale blue room and said, "Hey, I'll take her."

Helen said, "No, Annette, it's okay. Go back to bed. She'll be fine."

"No" I said, "please give her to me?" I just wanted a chance. Anna started to scream as though I was a complete stranger. As I sang a favorite hymn softly, I felt the grief and sorrow circled us. I needed God to help us both. Anna was still fussy and Helen returned to take her back. "Let me try," I begged. Anna and I cried together. Finally, she relented. After she fell asleep in my arms, I whispered, "Hey, sweet girl, I am your Mama, and this is our song, the one we'll always share. I am so sorry I haven't been there for you. But I love you, and we will be all right, I promise." It was a breakthrough night. That little girl was mine. Once I claimed her, she accepted me. Bill did not want me to get up each night so he assumed the role of transport. He understood that I wanted to be her comforter—that she gave me a purpose greater than walking again.

Our relationship is full of the complexities of any mother and daughter, but there's something unspoken that we both honor. While she obviously doesn't remember her birth, a longing for it to have been different resides in her as well. It seemed an unfair burden that her entrance in the world coincided with my loss. I've asked her if she would like to choose another birthday. "No, Mom," she says. "It is my birthday, and honestly I can separate it." She's not afraid to be sad when we talk about it, and a few times she has come to me in tears saying she wishes it never happened. That is when I know that being at the foot of the cross is just as excruciating as being on it. I want to take her pain for her, but I can only hold her in my arms.

Bill perceives Anna's strength as defiance but, underneath it, I know that it's a mask for the deep sorrow that she had to be "the one." Will my injury be the thorn in her side? My therapist, Alison, said no. That Anna had the inner self to transcend this. Anna joined me in therapy— Alison suggested we draw pictures together. She offered little instruction, just handed us paper and crayons. When Anna was in pre-school, she was already the smartest girl in our home. Once finished, she handed Alison her finished masterpiece. She had drawn two mountains. I was on the top of one and she was on top of the other. "Annette," Alison said, smiling, "You see this? Anna is going to do just fine!"

Natalie does not remember our times together when I could still walk. Would it make a difference if she did? I wanted her to glimpse who I thought I might be. I have a warm collection of lovely memories with her, just the two of us. There were frustrations of course, when she would not sleep, which was often. We drove up to Maine when she was just a baby. She cried through the night as we took turns walking her up and down the inn's hallway. Finally she fell asleep between us. Bill looked at me exhausted and said, "Annette, remind me why we thought this was a good idea?" I had never seen Maine, and that is why we thought it was a good idea! And, I am so grateful we went because it was the last time I explored the rocky coast of Maine on two feet. The wonderful times picking flowers with her, or jumping in a pile of leaves, or taking her to music together classes far outweighed the new challenges of parenthood. But, she has no memory of any of it...of me as a young, fun, happy mother. The one who took her to classes at Sarah Lawrence because I did not want to be apart from her. She once sat in a college classroom with Professor Afzal, and now she is college bound. Recently, as she was nearing high school graduation, I tried to jog those memories of our walks to the park and the nature center when she was in a stroller. "You don't remember any of it, Nat?" She looked at my sad face and said, "It's okay, Mom. It doesn't bother me." Only Bill remembered who I was. It may be that, more than needing *her* to remember, *I* wanted to remember.

After my injury, the doctors were convinced that I would not be able to conceive again. My body had been thrust into menopause and they had the blood work to prove it. This was a blow to my femininity, but I decided not to intervene with what nature was doing. "Shut it down," I thought. "It's probably best." I was only 33 and it was not the thought of only two children that frightened me, it was menopause itself. I knew nothing about how my already disoriented body would act. Still in the discovery phase, my approach toward my health was completely holistic. Bill and I used natural methods of birth control. This decision was made partly due to my religious philosophy, but also because I didn't believe we could get pregnant again.

Two years on, I remember watching the clouds from our bedroom window. They were like giant cotton balls floating across the sky. As they billowed passed, two connected in such a way that made me picture a baby. I'd never before had a premonition, and I didn't speak a word of it, not even to Bill. But I knew that—somehow—we would have more children. A year later, we were pregnant.

"What if I die this time?" I asked my priest friend, Father Les.

"Of course you're scared," he said. "But I will pray for you." It would require more than prayer.

We consulted Nicole and Teri the nurses, now friends, who took care of me at Yale. They recommended an obstetrician who they said was perfect for me. Her name was Dr. Urania Magriples and she was a fit from the moment we met. My friends had filled her in on Anna's birth before our first meeting. She was confident that this pregnancy was going to go well, and she would see to it. It was a relief. This one is yours, I thought, and she was well equipped to take it on. In fact, during our first conversation she mentioned delivering babies in Africa. She made the trip almost every year. "They don't use any drugs," she said, "they just sit in the grass and have their babies like it's the most natural thing in the world." I wanted to meet these women. While I did not think I could have our baby outdoors I was nonetheless inspired. The pregnancy was issue-free. As my delivery date approached Urania sat me down and said two things, "Annette, I am going to be out of town two weeks before your due date, I don't think you will have the baby but I wanted you to know."

Hadn't I heard that once before? I sighed and tried not to be scared. She went on to say that she expected that after the birth, I would have some symptoms of post-traumatic stress and that she was ready for it. Ingrid was born when she was out of town, another little test, but I laughed at the irony. The next couple days I did have a big spike in my blood pressure. They got Urania on the phone to reassure me. "I fully expected your body to have a reaction. This will pass, Annette. You have to trust me."

Trust, what does it mean to trust? Trust her? God? The universe? Fate? I had to settle down. Blood pressure is just numbers, I told myself if she was worried, then I could be; but she was not. Our third child, Ingrid Anne was born on Father Les's birthday. An answer to prayer? He was relieved and came to meet her with a huge smile holding a big red stuffed dog which Ingrid slept with every night.

I chose "Ingrid" because I'd always loved Ingrid Bergman, but the name has another significance meaning "hero's daughter" in Norwegian. Given that Urania was not present to "catch the baby" the delivery could not have been less remarkable. In place of the epidural they offered a shot of narcotic that made me loopy. The doctor stood patiently at the foot of the bed and talked quietly to Bill. I interrupted them. "What is your name?" I asked. It was an Indian name; I could not pronounce it correctly so I asked one more time. "I'm sorry I didn't get that— can you tell me again?" He said it again, but it was time to push. "It is time," he said. Did he know what to do?

"Have you talked to Urania, doctor? Did she fill you in?" (I could not remember how to say his name.) "I am so sorry I just cannot remember your name!" I blurted out. Bill and the doctor laughed at me while repeating his name once more in unison. My first time on drugs...I guess it was hilarious. Bill had been less involved with the previous deliveries, but this time he cut the umbilical cord. This act of solidarity bonded him to Ingrid.

Our life began to take a new direction. The effects of such an easy childbirth convinced me that I was superwoman.

The next day Bill and I brought Ingrid home to our warm rambling farmhouse. Something new and good was happening. Ingrid's life felt like a miracle. The pregnancy even changed my body, bringing back proper bladder function. Once the path to new life was rebooted within me, very soon we were pregnant with Mia. She was healthy and beautiful, born on the morning of Christmas Eve 2004. This time Urania was there. It was exciting to watch her in action. Nothing fazed her. She was calm (and funny), and I relaxed in her presence. During delivery there was one slight blip. Urania looked at the monitor and calmly said, "Annette, lie on your side. I am not sure why but the baby's heart rate has dropped." She looked at the head about to crown, saw what the problem was and told me to push. Once out, she unwrapped the cord and showed it to me. "Look at this, Annette. Look at how beautiful the umbilical cord is." I had never seen one and since the nurses had Mia with them I stopped to really admire it. She was right, it was spectacular. The color was one I've never seen — not even in a box of 64 Crayolas. It was a translucent whitish purple, but there was something more. I've never *seen* childbirth, Bill has of course, and this was my first glimpse at what happened inside of me while Mia was growing. I paused to consider how this organ somehow, miraculously, nurtured our baby over the last nine months. I said a silent "thank you." There are moments of awe and wonder that we do not want to break away from and this was one of mine. We took Mia home on Christmas Day. Santa had already visited, but the best gift we have ever received was in our arms. With four daughters our family was complete. I was still trying to walk, and anxious to get back in shape, but life was blessing us.

After Bill and I were married for a year, I decided to find my biological mother. My life with Bill had such a synchronized rhythm, I knew that no matter what I faced, it would be fine, and that even if the worst were true, I could handle it.

I began simply with the phone book. Before Betty and Bill Fenwick officially adopted me, they fostered me as an infant and my sister Patti remembered the unusual last name I'd arrived with. There were three people in the Chicago vicinity to call and it happened that they were all related to my mother, Connie. I found her sister Gina first. She did not recommend that I contact Connie directly but agreed to meet me, along with their mother Claire (my biological grandmother), at P.J. Clarke's in Chicago's Lincoln Park. I walked with Bill to the restaurant, nervous and excited. They recognized me immediately. It was obvious from their reserved reaction, they shared my apprehension. It was early, and the bar was quiet. We sat at a corner table. I think they questioned what I wanted from them and made it clear that, although they trusted me enough to share Connie's story, there would be no direct contact with her. Connie, they insisted, was too fragile to meet me. The family had endured many tragedies, the most dramatic being the death of their father when Connie was only in eighth grade. Claire was left to raise three young children alone. Being the eldest, Connie quickly immersed herself in the duties that once belonged to her father. She cleaned, did all of yard maintenance, and fixed whatever was broken. She shouldered the burden with her mother, but it was a storm that never fully passed. The family would not have the same happiness again.

And you could sense it—that they survived, they smiled, but there was pain behind the smiles. When she got pregnant with me, in the late 60's (and out of wedlock), it became the family secret. Over the years, Connie remained single. Instead she lived at home with her widowed mother until she was diagnosed with a brain tumor. When I met Gina and Claire in 1996, Connie was doing well, meaning she was able to sustain her work and home life. Their fear was that I would disrupt the delicate balance that everyone had worked so hard to achieve, especially Connie. Knowing that this beautiful woman never married and instead stayed to care for her mother was all I needed to know. Her younger brother Michael never knew that I existed until I surprised his wife, Janet, with a phone call. And, because Gina and Claire did not inform them that I was attempting to contact Connie, finding out was a source of more tension within the family. Janet was gracious and supportive of me from the very beginning. She understood why I would want to know Connie, and she offered to help. But I needed to respect the wishes of Gina and Claire. They had lived with and knew Connie best. It would not be right to do otherwise, and so I stayed away. When we had said all that could be said in only one afternoon, I expressed my appreciation to them. I sensed they were still worried that I might not respect their request to leave Connie alone, but it was never an issue. They had given me a glimpse of who my mother was as a young girl, and then as a woman. If they could not fully embrace me, it was not personal. The family had endured too much already.

Over the years, I mostly kept in touch with Janet, who never failed to send me a Christmas card with updates on her life with Michael, and their two boys. When Connie was sick, and her death imminent, it was Janet who rallied the family on my behalf. This time, I was the wounded one, but did I want to meet Connie in my wheelchair? *Yes*, I did. We gathered Natalie and Anna for a road trip to Chicago. It was fall of 2001, and the color on the trees was brilliant, but melancholy. The seasons illuminate death and renewal each year, and this would be Connie's last. Before we left, I sent Connie a bouquet of roses—34 in all—one rose in gratitude for each year of my life. I was thankful she had me, and now her courage and beauty would be passed down for generations. The family was going to prep her for our arrival, and although I was somewhat apprehensive about the visit, I hoped it would be a warm and loving reunion.

A real fantasy was about to come true. I'd imagined our first meeting hundreds of times. She would lovingly ask me all sorts of questions about how I'd grown up, my likes and dislikes, and if I'd been happy. And then she'd tell me of how much she had longed for me. Although I knew Connie's story, or parts of it, it still did not resonate until I saw her in the hospital bed. She was lying down in the bed, looking toward the window, her head partly shaven. She was still beautiful, but a lonely woman with regrets and deep sorrow. I wheeled in with only Bill. She turned her weary gaze at me and said, "Hey, you."

"Do you know who I am?" I asked her. She nodded.

She didn't ask about my life, but looked from me to Bill and told me, "You're luckier than I ever was."

I felt only empathy for this beautiful, fragile woman, whose life had held its share of tragedy. When she'd become pregnant with me, she'd been in denial about her situation; clearly, it was not in her nature to consider a life to be "a tumor growing inside."

I learned that she had once been a concert pianist. That she'd so idolized Leonard Bernstein and used to bake a cake on his birthday each year. She'd also played piano part-time at fancy lounges. I don't know for sure, but think she may have met the man who would become my father at one of them. (I like to think that she passed her musical passion on to me.)

Connie asked that we return the next day and to bring our girls. I felt that this was a small victory, and hoped it meant that she liked me. Her sensitive nature was revealed when she saw

Natalie and Anna. "They're beautiful! And you're so lucky," she beamed. I reminded her that they owed their beauty, in part, to *her*. When it was time for us to go, Connie let out an almost visceral cry of "Anna!" and stretched out her arms to our baby girl. We came back so that she could take one last look before we said goodbye.

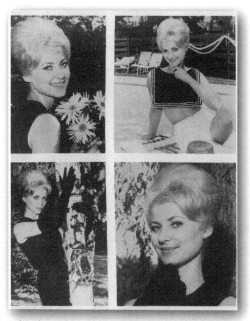

My birthmother Connie's glamour shots. She was also crowned Lilac Queen in her town.

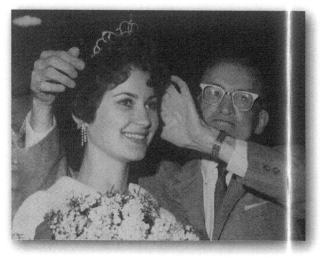

Surgery Hope

DURING THOSE EARLY YEARS AFTER the injury, it was my unwavering belief that the only life for us was one in which I was walking. So we vigorously pursued different rehab options around the country. And we decided that it was important to have the girls with us. Those sweet little faces kept me going after a tough day of therapy. Natalie was five and Anna two when we began traveling the 17-hours between New Canaan and Washington University in St. Louis, Missouri, where I underwent therapy for months at a time. Nat's kindergarten teacher expressed concern at her missing part of the school year. In hindsight, I wonder if it was a selfish choice. When they look back, will the girls understand that we had the best of intentions?

I once read an essay in *New Mobility* magazine called, "The High Costs of Walking." Many individuals with spinal cord injuries spend their remaining resources, compromise family life, and give up all else in pursuit of the dream. Now, after many years of effort, I ask myself if we did the best thing for our family. The moments of hope and promise enticed us, but ended unfulfilled.

The article brought me back to that time, when we traveled back and forth to St. Louis, and then to Baltimore, in hopes of finding that one physician. Every patient in search of a cure longs to find a doctor who shares their commitment and resolve, but it is rare, especially with the way medicine is practiced today. Doctors are busy, bombarded with paper work, told to only see patients for the allotted 15 minutes. It's not that they don't want to go the distance. There's too much for them to do. And, there is the emotional element. How can they travel the road of victories and defeats with everyone?

But, we found such a doctor. Dr. Cristina Sadowsky understood my passion and, with her guidance, we devised a plan to move forward. It was she who lovingly told me to get out of my head and enjoy sex again. She was right about that, so I had full confidence that she would see enough promise in the strength I had already recovered and strategize a way to functionally use my weak, spastic legs. After assessing my progress for a couple of years, and waiting for me to finish a pregnancy, she firmly believed the obstacle to my improvement was getting my feet flat. This would require surgery — only I wanted nothing to do with it. Was there another way?

We tried a series of casts. My feet were stuck in plantar flexion (pointing down) and, to walk properly, they needed to have more dorsal flexion. The goal was to enable my foot to stretch to 90 degrees, which meant heel on the ground. The Achilles was so tight, it only allowed for a few degrees of movement each week, and we had a way to go. The entire procedure would take eight weeks or more with a cast change each week. My Achilles tendon rebelled in the casts. They spasmed all night long, shaking inside the fiberglass, and making sleep impossible. There was too much friction. I could feel a pressure wound developing. One night, in intense discomfort, I sought to take the cast off myself. "Is it worth it, Bill? If I get a sore, it's a major setback. I risk infection, and my sensation is not good enough to trust what is happening inside there. I have to get them off!"

Bill came back with, "I agree, Annette, but wait until we're at the doctor's. They'll take the casts off." I started to claw at the cast. I dug a small hole near the heel to peer inside, but the cast was too thick.

"Bill," I pleaded. "Help me!" We had no tools, except a hacksaw. He dutifully went to the garage.

"Are you sure you want to do this? What if I cut your leg?"

"You won't," I assured him. "I can feel the vibration enough to tell you when to stop." And he proceeded to cut both casts off my legs without so much as a scratch. The doctor was NOT happy with us. Even so, we tried another set of casts with extra padding, and Bill and I went out to purchase a cast saw just in case. Days later, I looked at Bill and pointed to my casts.

"Oh, no," he said.

"Yes. Go get the saw." This treatment was not going to work.

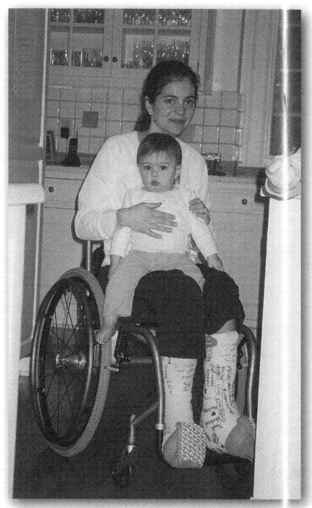

In my casts from Achilles' surgery with Mia.

We discussed the surgical option again. "I am really fine with it, but do we have to use anesthesia?" The narcotics worked fine for childbirth. They looked at me like I was insane to suggest this — but that was my mental block, the medicine. The lawsuit was still in discovery phase, and it was unclear exactly what happened. Each side had only theories. A part of me feared that the medications paralyzed me. They sent me to meet with an anesthesiologist. She had long blond hair, a quiet demeanor, and sharp blue eyes. She was aware of what happened with the epidural.

"Don't be afraid," she said. "Nothing will happen to you under my care, I promise."

"Don't say that," I said, "it's not fair to you, you can't know what will happen, and I understand that."

"No," she insisted, "I mean it. I will not let anything happen."

I liked her confidence. But what if? She wouldn't hear of it. She would see me through the surgery. The morning I went in, I was calm.

She stood over me and said, "How do you feel?"

I returned her confidence and said, "I feel ready to walk again."

Her eyes were the last thing I remember until I woke up. A week after they took my casts off from surgery, I stood with my walker. For the first time in five years, my feet were able to stay flat on the ground, and I took ten unforgettable steps. Tears poured down my face as I recalled what it felt like to feel the weight of my own body. I thanked my bony legs for not letting me down. "Bill, it is going to happen!" I screamed. He sprinted over to hug me. Our dream would become reality.

In order to keep the momentum, we travelled to Baltimore. Cristina had an intense therapy plan. Despite the hours of water therapy, electrical stimulation and unweighted-gait training, my legs did not get stronger. We drove up to Boston for another opinion. I walked twenty steps in the walker. The doctor shook his head, but said nothing. This proved just enough for the doctor to determine why I wasn't progressing. Finally he spoke, "It has been years now, and the nerve function that's been restored is most likely all you'll get. Your walking will never be functional and should you continue, you run the risk of a greater injury."

So that was it? Did he just say I would never walk again? We thought it would just take more time. We needed to believe, follow the dream, think positive. We explored alternatives, and spent even more money. Was it worth it? Here's what I learned: that denial is powerful. And, we met some pretty fabulous people. Good people are always worth it. Each time we pulled up to the hotel in St. Louis, the staff stood outside, waiting for us (so it seemed) ready to greet the girls with cookies and balloons. It never felt like we were staying at a foreign place, but a home away from home. And they shared in my dream to walk again. The same was true of Baltimore. One year we were there for the Fourth of July. I was working hard, but had the day off. We ate blue crabs with Old Bay Seasoning in the afternoon then walked down to the harbor and watched the night sky light up. There was no music to accompany the display, but the 1812 Overture played in my head. I wanted to turn it up, so everyone could hear it with me. I am going to walk again, I told myself as I looked at the girls. But this moment, right now, feels complete.

More Loss

My own Mom, Betty, died in late July of 2007. We went to Chicago for her funeral. Natalie, Anna, Ingrid, and Mia joined us. The most difficult part was seeing Dad. He quietly walked around the funeral home, warmly embracing the family and friends who came to acknowledge her life. He looked as though he was missing something, an appendage, and he was. Mom was his best friend, the one who promised almost 60 years earlier to be at his side for a lifetime. He was sorrowful, but radiated a profound peace. A year before her death, Mom was diagnosed with dementia. It progressed to the point where Dad took care of her full-time. It was his joy to care for her always, but his health issues were not improving, and his fervent prayer was that she would never have to live a day without him. In that way, God fulfilled his wish. Mom never lived one day without her loyal, trusted companion, and he was able to let her go.

I was 40-years-old and 16 weeks pregnant with our first boy at the funeral. At the casket, I silently thanked Mom for giving me the boy she knew we so wanted. During our last phone conversation, she hadn't been sure who I was, and after the call I wept. I still needed her to know me, to care about my life; she was the only mother I had, and our relationship felt unfinished.

We came home from Chicago emotionally drained. And yet, we were looking ahead, excited about our first baby boy. Two weeks after Mom's funeral, almost to the halfway mark of the pregnancy, I began to bleed bright red blood. We called Urania and she told us to rush to the hospital. Once there an ultrasound revealed that our baby was dead; had actually died a week earlier. The doctors needed to take me to surgery, to stop my bleeding, but first asked if we wanted to see the baby before they wheeled me away. Yes, we did. They brought him to us in a small, yellow, plastic tray. We blessed him, and with that our baby boy was gone. They wheeled me into the operating room. When I woke later, my heart was empty. "Bill, what happened?" He shook his head.

We'd left home in such a hurry, the girls knew something wasn't right. Natalie and Anna, and even Ingrid, were old enough to recognize that. Five-year-old Ingrid was the most visibly upset. She cried, "Where's the baby?"

To say that God wanted the baby, or that the baby was now with God, did not console me. Would it console her? Terrible, unthinkable things happen. This was one of those things. "The truth is, Ingrid, we don't know what happened, and Dad and I are heartbroken, too." That was all I could say to my little blond sweetheart. Mia stood like a pale statue in the doorway. She was only three.

Bill fell into a depression. He'd lined up framed football jerseys against the nursery wall that we'd planned to paint blue. He'd pulled his train set out of the attic. He'd planned and dreamt of the day when he would play catch in the yard with the son who would share his name. It was not to be.

When our little boy died, I needed to understand what happened with God all over again. Prayer did not console me. The girls were the only light penetrating our darkness.

Bill dealt with his pain silently. It was the start of his downward spiral. Despite not being overtly religious, he shares a special relationship with the Blessed Virgin Mary. She literally stood outside his office window—a small concrete statue that we found on the side of a local road, and claimed for our own not long after I was injured. While in my "healing phase" we took a drive down Route 1 in Wilton and saw her the first time. "Bill, stop," I said.

"Oh no, Annette, I am not getting that statue," he insisted.

"But I feel it belongs to us."

"Annette, really, I am not stopping the car." We drove away. Weeks later we were on that same road and she was there. I looked at Bill, and he smiled as he drove on. The next time we saw her, he turned to me and said, "Annette, if she is still there the next time we come this way, we will get her." A month passed, and she was still there, her arms at her side, with open palms while her feet squashed the head of the serpent. Bill kept his word. And she has a home wherever our pilgrim road takes us.

Whatever was happening inside of Bill he would later call "the perfect storm." There was no way for him to relieve his frustrations, so he tried taking it out in the financial markets. It didn't happen with purpose or thought; he just began to wage some kind of private war in his office. Something in our home did not feel good. After losing our baby boy, a karmic shift occurred. You could sense it, but could not name it precisely. Still, a feeling of hopelessness prevailed.

We got pregnant again right away—not on purpose. The idea that I was a fertile person never sank in. Ingrid was conceived after my doctors had diagnosed me as having entered menopause. Mia was born because my body was working normally again, but that would surely be it, or so we thought. I made efforts to avoid pregnancy, but they were (clearly) not sufficient. It was a terrible feeling to have to defend it all the time. This time, I was pregnant with another little girl. At our 14-week appointment, the technician did an ultrasound, left the room, and promptly returned with the doctor. I knew something was wrong. Dr. Magriples performed a second ultrasound. The baby's hung head down in the birthing position with no heartbeat. Urania shook her head before saying it. "I am sorry, Annette."

The tears were burning my face. "Please take it out now," I cried. "I don't want to see the blood." They moved me to the operating room quickly. The anesthesiologist could not put me under fast enough. I looked into her blue eyes and said, "Please, I want to be out for a long time." My head, always crammed with thought, went quiet as they prepared me for surgery. I remember the doctor who was about to perform the D&C saying to me, "It could have been worse."

"Yes," I acknowledged. It could have been worse. And I drifted off into a deep sleep.

After allowing me time to grieve, Dr. Magriples called me at home. The baby had Trisomy 14, a genetic anomaly that was incompatible with life. Had the pregnancy continued, it would indeed have been worse. I took the phone outside on the balcony to speak with her. It was cold, and everything looked dead. I faced the statue of the Blessed Virgin as we spoke.

"Do not get pregnant again," she said. Her tone was matter of fact, I was worried that she was upset with me, that she was giving up on me or thinking that my body was old and tired. "The physical complications are too great, Annette." She added, "Please don't do this to yourself because of a belief system." She loved me like a friend, and cared enough about my being there for our daughters to say something. She was one of the finest doctors I knew. I trusted her. I did not know what to do. The conversation ended with tears. Overcome with grief, there was no way for me to wrap my head around what happened or even consider what to do next.

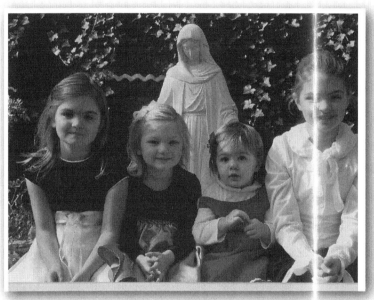

Four girls (Anna, Ingrid, Mia and Natalie) with
the statue of the Blessed Mother.

The Lawsuit

~⌒

WHEN WE FINALLY WENT TO court to seek damages for my injury, the Stamford courthouse lobby was being remodeled. Ironically, this meant it was not wheelchair accessible. And yet the word *JUSTICE* loomed over us, engraved near the ceiling. Justice. What did that mean for us?

Desmond Tutu once said, "I am willing to forgive you for stealing my pen, after you give it back." I think he was referring to how limited we are in our ability to forgive. I felt I had already forgiven: I just wanted my legs back, but that was not something the lawyers could give. Money hardly compensates for that type of loss, but that is how the system works. You wouldn't think it, but there are formulas for these things.

The unknown component is pain and suffering, and at the time of our litigation, the state was trying to put a cap on that. Our attorneys asked that I testify in front of a committee to discuss the particulars of my case. It was 2005, and Mia was just a tiny baby. We went to the courthouse in attempts to appeal to the panel's most basic human instincts. Yes, life can change in an instant, it can happen even in a place that is supposed to heal you, and no one is immune. Holding Mia in my wheelchair, I was living proof.

Justice does not always happen in court. But it is hard to calculate the loss of functioning legs. What about accompanying bone loss, bathroom issues, infections, and the way that people look at and treat me differently now? Once I'd observed the inner workings of the legal system for a while, I held no illusions. The attorneys on both sides of medical malpractice cases work together frequently. Bill and I spent hours in depositions, sitting between opposing legal teams who joked with each other easily, and on a first-name basis. Then they fired off questions. It was as if they asked the same question in a new way each time, to get me to say something different. What I had to say was simple. I walked into the hospital a healthy young woman about to give birth. I never walked out. But the chess game they were playing was in motion long before our case came up for review. As different tragedies occur, only a few variables change. Each year the hospital has a number of cases; the accused and the plaintiffs change, but the lawyers on both sides follow a well-worn script, and their game is the same. Sometimes one side captures the queen, but there is never a checkmate. It's hard to discern how lawyers feel about their clients; they see so much pain and suffering. But justice is not the ultimate end. And maybe that's because there is no such thing. If you receive what is equal to what you have lost, is that just? Having observed their interactions over many years, I've concluded that the primary objective for both sides is to stay in the game, to continue making money for the firm—and for themselves—for years to come. That's not to say that there aren't cases that settle in favor of the plaintiffs, but if there is justice, it serves the legal profession first.

The lawsuit was not our bid to buy a luxury home in Bermuda. We only sought the opportunity to work toward walking again. Therapy for life seemed reasonable. But what about Bill? He'd run a very successful business before taking on the Herculean task of being my sole caregiver. Why was there was no avenue to pursue his losses? The lawyers dismissed him.

The lawsuit took six long years to settle. It went all the way to jury selection. Then, the day before the trial was set to begin, the hospital offered a settlement. Sadly, the attorney who'd cared the most about us died during the years of depositions and discovery. He'd been the family attorney for the Rosses since Bill's birth. If he were there to advise us, we might not have settled. Surely, we would have benefitted from his counsel. What remained of our legal team was a group of talented lawyers who were ready to move on from our case. It was in their interest to settle. Bill did not agree. But I was ready. More years of litigation did not interest me. I wanted the focal point of our lives to shift away from tragedy. It seemed like a waste to continue, but Bill felt we should put it in front of the jury and let them decide.

Before a trial begins, the judge decides what a jury will be allowed to hear during testimony. Our judge ruled against what we thought were key pieces of evidence. The lawyers on our team were trying to figure out ways to work around his decision, but at the time of jury selection, it was not clear how they would proceed. Medical malpractice is as complex as criminal law. When the evidence is presented, a juror would expect to hear all of the evidence but the judge holds some of the cards. As the date for our trial drew closer, I asked to speak to the judge myself. I wanted him to see me. I wanted to ask him in person why he was ruling out such crucial evidence. It was then that I found out I was not allowed to discuss my case with the judge—that is why people hire lawyers. It was also then that we realized we had lost faith in them and their ability to go all the way for us. Should the jury award me a high settlement, it was explained that the appeal process could take us into Natalie's college years. Natalie in college…it was years and years away.

Given what happened next, I see that Bill was right. That we planned poorly. That our agreeing to settle before he felt the legal process had served us had a very negative effect on him. The part that I could not let go was not monetary, but how completely the process dismissed what happened between a doctor and her patient. Doctors take an oath to first do no harm. Did it matter that it was unintentional? Shortly after my injury, when I'd been transferred to Yale, the anesthesiologist came to see me there. Standing at the end of my bed she said, "I do not know what happened. I am sorry." We both began to cry, but before I could say a word or comprehend her presence at my bedside, she was ushered out of the room by a group of physicians. After that, we were never allowed to speak. She'd tried to approach me during jury selection, but was kept at a distance. She even followed us home once. (Bill thought she was spying on us, but I suspected that she just wanted to talk to me.) Years went by and we sat across a courtroom. What she and I needed to resolve had nothing to do with a settlement.

I wanted to free her from her burden. There were many emotions that surfaced when I saw her, but none of hate. She had not intended to change my life forever that night. Doctors are capable of many human failings. There was no doubt that she, too, had suffered. During the years of litigation, we heard that her husband died. I never met him, but mourned him. It could not have been easy for her. I knew that nothing short of full use of my legs as they once were would satisfy me, but I could still make peace with her. We should have been able to speak the words held in for so long. The judicial system should have allowed for it, or even supported it, but it didn't. And, so I learned what really happens when you go to court and, to be fair, both parties leave wishing it were different.

I've interacted with many doctors since 2000, most of whom initially ask me why I'm in a wheelchair. Their responses have varied, but only one apologized. He was someone new I was consulting, and when we spoke, he pulled up a stool to sit directly in front of me and asked, "What happened to you?" He listened intently to my story. "You have got to be kidding me," he said.

"I'm not kidding." I half smiled, "It was not my lucky night." I said lightly.

He slowly set his gloves down, and hugged me. "I am so sorry." He meant it. And I felt better. No doctor involved in my injury ever took responsibility for what happened. In the humanity of this man's response, I felt a collective apology.

Once everything was finalized, Bill and I agreed that a portion of the compensation from the case should be used to reestablish his business. If the law did not see fit to compensate him, I did. It was only fair after everything he'd sacrificed for me. One night at dinner, a friend said to me, "You know, Annette, people often make financial decisions that are not in their best interest."

What an odd thing to say. "What on earth do you mean?" I asked. He went on to explain that emotions often get in the way of good business sense. I kept thinking about his observation long after dinner. Was this a premonition? I often looked for "signs" and thought that, more than once, God put a person on our path to offer us guidance. But this hadn't resonated as a message from God, at least not right away. I couldn't connect the dots. Nevertheless, the conversation proved to be prophetic. The financial decisions we made in the aftermath of the lawsuit came from guilt, despair, and false hope. To put it in football terms, as Bill did so frequently, we fumbled the ball, and our team did not recover it. Our friend was like a messenger whose advice we could not hope to understand at the time.

Bill uses sports as a metaphor instead of God for everything—with our girls as well. He used to make them run around our property and time them with a stopwatch. "It's for discipline," he'd say. They rolled their eyes in annoyance but admitted, behind his back, that it was kind of endearing. "Girls," he'd say, "We are a team. And you can't let your team down." The gospel according to Bill is that every person benefits from playing on a team. He fails to see that somehow I have managed to be the most disciplined person in the family without it. It takes discipline to manage my weight without the benefit of walking and discipline to maintain a commitment to prayer in such a busy household, but that's one argument I won't win, which is fine.

But he's right that we truly are a team. Oddly enough, it was because of sports that Bill learned to pray. Whenever he lost a ball in the yard he prayed to find it. The same was true on game day. If there was rain, he invoked God to have the sun shine by kick off. He told me he did not miss church as a child, but always believed that life held meaning and purpose and that human beings were mysteriously connected. He once saved the life of someone who had come to complete despair, although that is his story to tell. When someone calls upon Bill for help, he shows up. I say that I know more about *religion* — and I do — but in truth where my faith ends is where his begins.

There's a great line in a Woody Allen film: "Is a memory something we have gained or something we have lost?" The answer is: both. I feel too young to have only memories sustain me.

My internal calendar marks the years as "before" and "after." Our former life feels more and more like a dream. All joy has not ceased, but unadulterated joy falls in the category of "before." It may be the loss of innocence that made the greatest impact. This includes the surety of my faith. It was not just the walking and running that was lost, but the understanding of how God worked. Although it was terribly naive to think I ever grasped the workings of God. My faith was once simple like Bill's when he was in search of a lost ball. That is what Dad said, "Have the faith of a child." To do that, you cannot ask too many questions. I once asked him what he would ask God once he got to heaven. "Not a thing, Annette, my cup will be full." That simple faith is hard won; it comes after years of prayer, discipline of the mind, and probably a fair share of disappointments. Dad would tell me to relish the happy memories, and make more of them. "You forget, Ann, that so much of it is up to you, you do not have to wait on God."

Perhaps there were missed opportunities within our tragedy we could not embrace. God may have been calling us, but did we hear Him? Should we have started an organization to help others? Did we use what happened to us for good? It always seemed that life was throwing us another pitch.

Life in a wheelchair is a series of small, monotonous details. You cease to move in a fluid, natural way. Consider the extra steps associated with my leaving the house: there's the requisite stop at the bathroom, transfer to the car, disassembly and loading of the chair, various adjustments, and off we go…only to do it all over again at the other end, this time in reverse. Even fifteen years on, I'm still not used to it. But you adjust. It all comes down to compromise.

Chair or no chair, my kids expect me to be a mother. I'm the sous chef for every meal, and the "go to" parent when they're searching for soccer cleats, writing a paper, or need help printing out a homework assignment before rushing out the door. Two of our girls play soccer. I try, but don't make it to every game. Sometimes, it's just easier if Bill takes them and avoids the inevitable, "Mom, you are going to make us late again," and then, "Where will we park, how close is the field, is there an accessible bathroom?" There's usually a portable outhouse at the games, but rarely (if ever) an accessible one. I recoil at the clumsiness—and sometimes filthiness—of situations I've encountered.

When the girls are inconvenienced because of me, I feel a tremendous sense of guilt. Picture your day from the vantage point of a wheelchair. Would you be able to leave your home without assistance? Sit with friends at a live performance? Access public transportation? How difficult would it be to enter and navigate the places you go each day on your own? (Do the doors open in or out? Is there a step up to go inside?) If an elevator is out of order, how would you feel about transferring out of the chair and onto the ground to get where you need to be?

Envision the machinations involved in using an airplane restroom. And the eye rolling and huffing of your fellow passengers. (Passengers who, by the way, tend to use the restroom way more frequently than I do—I've conducted an unofficial study of this phenomenon.) Imagine your response to the suggestion that I received from one flight attendant to "consider wearing a diaper next time" so as not to inconvenience the crew. That indignity cost the airline a free flight. Not the sort of windfall I'd been looking for.

The Americans with Disabilities Act (ADA) is a shockingly recent piece of legislation (established in 1990) that 'prohibits discrimination and ensures equal opportunity for persons with disabilities in employment, State and local government services, public accommodations, commercial facilities, and transportation." Many businesses take liberties and skirt ADA requirements. I applaud my friends who get out there and advocate for greater accessibility, because it benefits all of us and, in time, things do change. But not nearly quickly enough.

Having a disability made me feel more vulnerable, in part to other people, but even more so to the state and to institutions. We've all got stories about the arbitrary nature of the Department of Motor Vehicles. In my case, I'd gone there to have a hand-controlled break installed in my car. The DMV wanted me to have the model that included a manual gas pedal as well. I explained that I had use of my right foot—in fact used t daily in driving—but agreed to the second hand-held device. (I know my limitations, and figured it would be a help if my right foot grew fatigued on a long drive.) But when I was told that they would add a directive my license, limiting my permission to drive only that particular car, I balked. I told them, again, about my functioning right foot. They passed me along to a 21-year-old DMV employee to assess my range of motion. He was not a doctor, nurse or therapist. He had zero training in how to evaluate my ability or deficiency. Did he have the authority to tell me my foot was not good enough to use? It scares me to think of how easily I was labeled, and summarily had my rights limited. But, it happens all the time.

The reality for quads and paras is this: once you have a wheelchair, you are dependent. Perhaps you need help in order to eat, or to shower, or only when your tire goes flat. There are varying levels of dependency. Now that I use a wheelchair full-time, I sometimes feel unfamiliar, isolated, and a burden, maybe not to society at large, but certainly to my family.

There are certain books you can read more than once. Upon each reading, something new is illuminated. The first time I read Kafka's *Metamorphosis*, it was fantasy. The second time, it saddened me. The third and most recent time (I was injured by then), the end of the book angered me. One can make the assumption that the man, or creature, dies. He has been left in his room, alone, abandoned and rejected. The family views his emaciated body with pity, then, as if he were nothing, leaves it for someone else to dispose of. Freed from their burden, his family begins life anew. What if my family was happier freed from the burden of me? As much as they love me, the chair accompanies me, the bathroom concerns, and the extra labor. I think I'm worth it because I believe I would be there for them, but I do think about it. As Bill has said, "it is not a death sentence, but life in prison." He is the person whose life changed the most dramatically.

I have often said to the girls, "Oh, I wish you'd known me before I was hurt." I wish we could have taken walks on the beach, and hiked in the woods, but it is Bill I wish they could have known. His happiness was contagious, infectious, and everyone had more fun just because he was there. That changed. He changed. If I told him I was sorry, it would upset him. I know I did not cause this, but I am sorry, always.

And the girls will never know the person who married Bill. We tell them the stories and show them the pictures. Instead, they will remember the day I threw my shoes away.

I love shoes. Let me rephrase: I loved shoes. When I was little I had two pairs of shoes. One pair of sneakers and a pair of brown lace-up "every day" shoes. When I worked and could afford to buy my own shoes, I found it fun. Never one to pull off a fancy high heel, I preferred more substantial styles like Mary Janes and wedges with thick, clunky heels. They were comfortable, eclectic, and interesting. The way I see it, feet take you places, but shoes take you there in style! One afternoon in 2006, my friend Danielle, a lovely college student who sometimes helped with the girls, surveyed my closet.

"What's the deal with all these shoes? You never wear them."

"Well, I like them," I explained, somewhat defensively. "They bring back memories of my being able to walk, and someday I might be able to wear them again."

"Annette, it's time."

"Oh no," I pleaded, "I'm not ready."

"Annette," she said indignantly, "You may very well walk again, but when you do, you'll want to buy new shoes! These will be outdated."

She started to dust off some boxes. It was like looking at the shoes of a dead person. We held a small ceremony—Danielle listening as I shared stories of my favorites, like the black, leather Mary Janes I'd so happily worn that magical month in Italy. Off they went to be donated. I hoped that some part of who I'd been when I last wore them would be passed along to their next owner.

To bolster my mood, I started to look for funky shoe websites. There must be plenty of shoemakers that I had yet to discover. The girls were too young back then to offer me fashion advice. (Today they have plenty to say!) But, they understood that I was sad the day Danielle left with my shoes from another lifetime.

Getting rid of my shoes was a form of acceptance. My life was different now, and that change was so profound it included what I wore on my feet. Because my feet are swollen to varying degrees (depending on the weather), I choose shoes that cover my entire foot. My feet are now also slightly purplish, and that embarrasses me. Today, I wear mostly lace up sneakers and short boots. In addition to being swollen, even on a warm day, my feet are cold because of the decreased circulation, so it helps if a shoe has a little insulation. I can easily find a pair of shoes for almost any occasion now, and I periodically try something new. This can lead to a sore on my foot, which discourages me. "It's only a shoe," I tell myself.

And yet, I acknowledge, I've been more fortunate than most. A friend of mine who was a quadriplegic fell out of his chair while reaching for something when his caregiver didn't show up. He lay on the floor, injured, for half a day before anyone came to his aid. His wound became infected, the infection became systemic, and he died. This wonderful man, so full of life. He'd gone on speaking tours across the country, offering inspiration to hundreds, maybe even thousands of people. He'd also been working on his second book. He believed he would walk again. When I learned of his death, I was stunned. That he'd died alone bothered me more than anything else. Many of his companions were no longer at his side. He had fewer friends. Maybe he glimpsed that this was his end. Mutual friends shared that he'd felt that life was becoming too burdensome; that he was done living. Despite all his dreams, he lost his will to live.

Another friend, also in a chair, but from multiple sclerosis, confided that she, too, felt increasingly isolated. Her family claimed that she was no longer competent to care for her grade-school children and fought her in court. The husband who left her once she became disabled used the severity of her condition to win custody. I remember the distress in her voice as she expressed her love for her children. What was her recourse? It doesn't take much to take children away from someone with a disability, even when it's wrong. Left on her own for much of the time, she grew too frightened at night to transfer herself into bed, for fear that one morning she'd wake to find she didn't have the strength to get out again. We were, both of us, trying to be the best mothers we could be for our children. The difference was that I knew my husband would never use my disability against me.

Bill was not perfect, I knew that even before I married him, but I loved him. And he was very familiar with my peccadillos, yet he loved me. He put up with the fact that I hate to drive even on a perfect weather day, even when I know where I am going, even if all is right with the world. I do not enjoy driving and he accepts it. Thankfully for all of us, he loves to drive.

But has always needed ways to escape the inevitable dullness that accompanies reality. It was a simple achievement when we were young, in Chicago. The challenge proved almost impossible once I was injured. After I had endured my worst times I needed everything else to go smoothly. Bill would later (and lovingly) describe feeling like I had him in a vice grip. He felt unable to give his best to anything. "You can't go coach football! You can't go hang out with your buddies! I need you here." Bill recognized that my obsessive behavior came from a place of inner turmoil. And, not wanting to make things worse for me, he stayed close. We had less conflict when he was home.

Even with so much capital being diverted to my care, and the inadequate lawsuit settlement, Bill attempted to make the numbers work. The rate of return necessary to keep everything moving forward stressed his business. I guess the injury was outside of his business plan, and he was angry, especially at the lost time, but voicing a silent protest. He didn't care. He sought authority over some piece of his life. Bill's inability to share his problems with me caused me to question everything. He was acting strange and I sensed something was up. I became like a cop following him around the house. Finally, he spoke. "Annette, I think we need to sell the house." Not once had I ever envisioned that I would end up in a wheelchair. Likewise, I never gave a second thought to the idea that we might one day leave our home. It's not the things you are afraid of that happen to you.

I felt a new feeling of powerlessness. It was different than how I felt when I first became disabled. We weren't helpless, but we didn't know what to do. I wanted Dad to fix it. To be little again and have him protect me from the awful things beyond my control. If he could have done it, he would have. Since he couldn't, I wished with all my being that I could instantly become more like him: a person with few expectations, but happy for everything that came his way.

The news that we needed to sell devastated me, yet somehow, Bill and I remained close. We had our talks into the late night hours, not about how we felt right then, but about his childhood memories. He talked about football, the green army men he played with on the Silvermine River, and when his dad took down the trees in the yard to make a field for him to play on. His more recent interactions with his father hurt him, their relationship was fractured because of things said and not said. Whenever Bill tried to discuss the things that mattered most, his dad changed the subject. So Bill reminisced about happier times. It kept us both distracted — off of any painful subjects. We became absorbed in the past. Me, from when I could walk, and he from even earlier. I feared I was losing him to his unhappiness because of my fear of change. I was adamant that we would not experience more loss. This was new territory for both of us, but it should not have been, it was just one more broken dream. Instinctively, and maybe for survival alone, he expressed to me how he felt. "The house is swallowing me up," he said. "I can't stand it."

I did not understand what he meant. "What does that mean, Bill, you are becoming the walls?"

"YES", he said. "I am not the person I was. I am not who I hoped I would be. I do not feel I belong here any longer."

"Then where do we belong, Bill? This was our dream, we have to fight for it." Bill was looking for something now, and it was the first time we were not on par with one another. If I gave in to him, was I letting him down? Maybe he needed me to be the strong one. It was hard to tell what he really wanted, and I could not stop thinking about our long walks in Chicago. What happened? It was like living someone else's story; this was not supposed to be us.

The culmination of years of his being housebound with me and my wheelchair worked fine for me, but not for him. He'd stepped away from his business to attend to my needs, and I allowed it. I requested his presence at every appointment. Had he not done so, would I have survived? In my mind, I would still be lost somewhere. And, so when it was time for us to say goodbye to a life I embraced, deep down I knew my injury was the catalyst that led up to it. Now Bill needed me to give as much as he had given. We have each loved quite imperfectly, and yet, when necessary we loved one another more than we loved ourselves. What does it mean to love? How much was I willing to give? But, we were losing our house...would have to move. No more novenas at the statue of the Blessed Mother. It was over. There was no place to vet my feelings. I was with Bill, no matter the repercussions. But it was not just us, it was us with our daughters, and I knew what was on the horizon for them.

Leaving Our Dream Home

⌒

WHEN WE MOVED INTO THE Pines, we remodeled what was already a stunning kitchen. (My idea.) I chose a distressed, sea-green tile with images from a German fairy tale. In the story, a poor fisherman catches an enchanted fish that offers the man a wish in exchange for its freedom. The fisherman wishes for a better home for himself and his wife. The fish grants the wish; the fisherman returns home to find their living conditions improved. The conversation continues. Each time, the fisherman asks for a grander place to live, and the fish continues to deliver. Eventually the wife demands to rule. The fish, ever generous, allows her to be King, then Emperor, and even Pope. But this is not enough for the wife. She greedily asks to become like God, and although her husband begs her to be content with what she already has, she insists. The waters rage, the mountains shake, and the fisherman makes this final request. "Go home," says the fish. "Your wife is sitting in her filthy shack once more." I wanted the tiles to remind me always to be content. Now I wondered, had I not been satisfied with our life? Was God teaching me a lesson?

Our home was being taken apart piece by piece, and rolled up in the rugs, nothing was coming to save us. Not the Virgin Mary, not a fairy godmother, a magical fish, not family or friends. I tried to tell myself that none of it mattered. Family was who we were, not the house. Our belongings were just stuff that could be purchased again at a later time, and blah blah blah. But I knew it was gone for good...like my legs, and our boy. Bit by bit we were forced to let go of nearly all the things that once signified stability. Now I tried to remember the girls sliding down the stairs on their mattresses. I tried to be happy that we had lived somewhere so beautiful.

The days prior to leaving were filled with a longing to believe that none of it was actually happening. Natalie wrote in her journal, "Sadness is a sign on your front lawn that says 'For Sale,' and life will never be the same." The sign did not sadden me as much as anger me. "Mom, is there anything you can do?" she asked, as though I had a magic wand. Fresh out of ideas, I had no way to shield her from the reality that this was no longer home. Natalie's sorrow was mine, but I was her mother, the adult who was supposed to console her. Notorious for not hiding my feelings well, they all knew how miserable I was. One frown or wrinkle of my brow and the girls know how I feel. They teased me for being able to notice at least 30 seconds before I spilled the tears. "Mom, are you going to cry? Please don't!" The home, our family, and our resolve to beat the odds with my injury were all wrapped up together, and they got lost together.

California represents coming home for Bill. His parents adopted him in Los Angeles. He claims it's in his DNA. After college (when his dreams of playing professional football failed to materialize), he headed West, angry and disappointed. For a while, he lived on the beach, partied too much, and worked some really odd, unfulfilling jobs. One day he took in the surroundings and said to himself, "Time could stop for me here. I might stay and never do anything else." But it was with that realization that Bill knew it was time to move on; a more serious life awaited. And good fortune smiled on him. A friend from high school who respected his intensity and commitment called with a job offer at Trout Trading Management Company (TTMC). He said yes, and it changed the course of his life. Turned out, he was as good a trader as they'd suspected. Eventually he met me and...

We told everyone that we planned a move to California for progressive rehabilitation, which was partly true, but in truth too much had happened. Bill said time and again, "Annette, we have to move, the dream for us here has died, it's over." He kept repeating it so it would take hold in my consciousness but I could not let go. At night, I wheeled outside to pray at the statue of the Blessed Virgin Mary, which sat in the courtyard outside Bill's office door. "Please Mary, help us save our home. I've lost my ability to walk, can we keep the house?" I stayed outside in the cold hoping to convince a statue that we needed our home. I was bargaining, and begging. Back inside, I said to Bill, "Our prayer will be answered. Somehow, we will figure out a way to stay." And we tried. But mostly we waited, thinking that something magical would happen. The "For Sale" sign was on the lawn, but we rejected some early bids on the house. Bill was right though. It was done. He felt he failed. I felt I did. Maybe we both did.

Over the years, I had gazed out the French doors onto the lawn and imagined a grand party to celebrate my walking again. At first it was a dream home we purchased. But, it also became our refuge, and I did not fail to appreciate every exceptional detail. With the boxes packed and numbered, I travelled slowly down the hallway that led to our master bedroom. The wallpaper was so beautiful. The flowers were a large, whimsical pale blue that looked like a gorgeous bouquet was splashed right onto the wall. It reminded me of walking toward Bill on our wedding day with a bouquet full of large pastel ranunculus and roses; my smile full of hope, love, and possibility. The paper was chosen with the intent of recapturing that lovely moment each time I entered our room. Flowers brought me back to a time of beginnings; when something so simple and beautiful could also be magical. The wallpaper was not merely decor, but an extension of what I wanted my world to look like; my *vie en rose*. But we were leaving now. Every detail meant something special to me; the reality was converting to merely a memory. Picking out the wallpaper, the rugs, and the fabric was a learning experience as well as a privilege, and mirrored how I felt at the time—completely in love. Our home was more than the stone walls and a shingled roof— it was the place where I imagined the girls' wedding receptions, and where we would share Thanksgiving and Christmas dinners for years to come and then hopefully grow old together.

As I took the stair climber down for the last time, I thought, "We will never have a home again." I kept my head down as we drove away. At the airport, our flight to California was delayed. We called Ann and George, "Come back and stay the night," they offered. "Yes! A fabulous idea," I thought. Leaving our friends and neighbors on Hemlock Hill was like cutting off our lifeline. They saw us through the hardest days of my injury, they listened over pizza and wine as I explained my therapies, and even if George (sometimes) had his eyes shut I knew he heard every word! They hoped, every bit as much as we did, that I would walk again. Ann and George and our other dear friends Melinda and Jeff became like family. I left my family once in Chicago. Did I have to leave my new family? Being with them made everything better. I wanted to stay there with them on Hemlock Hill, frozen in time. Sitting in the airport, I knew our home was no longer ours, and I wanted to go back to our friends, wake up, and find that it had all been a bad dream. But Bill said no, we would wait. I stared out the window to watch where the planes pulled up to the gate.

The longer it remained empty, the closer I was to pretending this was not going to happen. Had we gone back, I don't think I would have had the strength to board the plane.

San Diego

～

THE SOIL IN SAN DIEGO makes it difficult for trees to grow; they don't easily root. Maybe that's why it was hard for me—like a tree, I found it difficult to thrive there. The landscape in its varying shades of brown is not without beauty. But for someone who appreciates the change and flow of seasons and the magic wrought by abundant rain, the absence of vibrant colors and dry wind takes getting used to. To the distant east there are small mountains, and due west nothing less than the mighty Pacific Ocean. There are worse places to land. You rarely meet a native of San Diego, or even of California—everyone's from someplace else. Another reason you do not sense deep roots. It felt more like a great place to hide rather than build a new community of friends. I wasn't sure what was missing—the absence of trees, familiar faces, or the sense that I knew I was home, which felt like it was gone for good. Maybe it was the weather; it is almost *too* good. Think about a place where the sun shines nearly every day and the temperature varies by no more than 20 degrees. My personality is too melancholy for that. A gray sky in San Diego is a day off, a relief. If it rains *and* dips below 70 degrees, I indulge in the moodiness of a tasty stew by a fake fire. There is a tendency to feel guilty if you're not out making optimal use of the fair gentle breezes and clear blue skies. But for one acclimated since birth to the rhythm of winters turning to spring, and summers giving way to autumn, you count on it. Its absence leaves me disoriented, adrift, and off course.

To get through our first year there, I worked harder than ever before to strengthen my legs. Incorporating acupuncture into my routine proved immensely beneficial. I found the needles scary, but with regular practice, I overcame my fear. As my legs grew stronger, my balance improved, and by year's end—and with minimal help—I could stand! An extraordinary achievement. My dream to walk was back in focus. It didn't matter to me that I was ten years into my "after" life. (Having been cautioned by a fellow in a wheelchair that no one walks again after a decade in a chair, I refused to be derailed.)

In January 2010, as the milestone anniversary approached, Anna worried. "Mom, are you okay that it's been so long?" She was still sensitive to the fact that her birthday and my injury were forever merged. A part of me grieved privately, but it was a day to celebrate our beloved Anna, and we did, with cake, candles, and a song. You could see already she was resilient and very bright, but what impressed me most of all was her wisdom.

Anna was wise beyond her years. She proved that as a newborn. Was it because of what happened? It was impossible to know, but while it seems the verdict is still out as to whether I will rise to the challenges set before me, Anna, our sweet girl, has passed the test.

I once gave a talk that I titled, "The Weight of Hope." I never thought of hope as being light—like "the thing with feathers" in the Emily Dickinson poem. I had to *work* at hope. But on my tenth anniversary, hope came easily, and my vision of us walking on the beach, hand in hand, came back into full view.

I missed home, but otherwise felt inspired. The miscarriages were behind us. Bill was busy networking. I spent most days at Awakenings Health Institute, where the community of friends I established provided the sense of family that I longed for. And the incredible trainers I worked with gave me strength and added a richness to my life. They also opened up my thoughts about disability. Adam, my patient and loving acupuncturist, insisted that when I looked out at the world in all its madness, it was my choice as to what lens to view it through. And, utilizing a favorite surfing analogy, he coached me in the concept of riding over the waves that I encountered, biding my time and waiting until a better one came along. He empowered me. I stopped judging myself and, in doing so, stopped judging others.

Before I ventured out on my own, before life really started to happen to me, I had been very much like my parents. My lens was black and white; varying shades of grey were too unsettling. In every scenario, I wanted to know who was right and who was wrong. Life is easy that way. Now I see everyone through the lens of compassion, even when it hurts. When the sting of a slap caused me to flinch back in fear, I came back with "they know not what they do." Dad helped me form a conscience, firm ideals, and a moral compass. I just needed to lose the rigidity. Love exists outside of my small judgments.

When we sold The Pines, that wonderful old farmhouse provided us with the means to keep things going…for a while anyway. San Diego, was not home, but we all grew and were better for it. We were not strong yet, but came up for air for long enough to take a deep breath. During that year, I'd given it my all, and accomplished the best work I had ever done with my legs. And that may well have been the pinnacle of what I would achieve. But the lack of business connections in California stagnated any momentum for Bill. Instead he found a position back on the East Coast.

I saw not one reason to stay. And yet, one bright afternoon when I picked up the phone to call Alison, I surprised myself. As I sat outside by Seaside Market looking out over the ocean I said, "Alison, I miss home, but there's something—something I cannot even articulate—that I like about it here. Have I become so shallow that it's the weather?" She laughed and listened carefully. "It occurs to me, Annette, that this has been an important time for your family. That said, Bill needs to be secure with his work, but I cannot say which place will be better in the long run. It is a weighty decision, one with many implications for all of you."

Bill's opportunity did not require a move for him to do the job, but I wanted to go *home*. It was time to return to family and friends. Bill agreed because he thought being able to sit face to face with the new people he would be working with was crucial. We loaded a Yorkie, a bunny, four daughters, and ourselves into a white van and headed toward the sunrise.

I was more than ready to resume our old life, but it was different when we returned. Maybe we should have known that it would be. Our home wasn't ours any longer. Old friends were there, but our status had changed. They questioned what had happened to us. The girls' found that their classmates had formed new friendships in their absence. We weren't entirely comfortable with our new house—a rental that we'd secured sight unseen. It wasn't just two stories, but choppy, with stairs throughout the entire first floor. We had to build a ramp inside of the screened in porch which connected two levels of the house. The bathroom was on the lower level. In winter, the ramp had snow on the rails, often I would slide down quickly and let the door catch me on the other side. We had a year's lease, so tried to make it work regardless. The best part of that first year home was the sledding hill on the side yard. We had a terrific snowfall, and Bill proved quite creative with mounds of snow and a shovel. He built the perfect slope for the girls to ride down and at the bottom he piled up enough snow for a fort. The snow lasted well into March, maybe even April. But beyond the snow-filled winter, we couldn't find our groove again. Almost upon our arrival, the business venture started winding down, layoffs occurred and, of the five initial employees, only Bill and the owner remained. The owner felt more comfortable returning to his original job in the city and decided to call it quits. Because Bill had worked for himself for the majority of his career, he had no stamp from a big Wall Street firm, which isolated him.

Should we head back to California? It was tempting, but another 3000 mile move was daunting. We stayed and Bill, who had just found his smile again, sunk back into a depression. He spent the majority of his time watching *The Walking Dead*. He was so engrossed with the zombies that it irritated him when he was interrupted. "I just want to see this one part! Can I have a moment's peace?" I suppose it was the perfect show to depict how he was feeling. This time I called George. Bill needed a friend, someone he could trust, and a person who believed in him. He also needed to get out of the house. George made Bill a priority, and for a time was the only friend who called regularly to check on him. They went for coffee, and sometimes grabbed lunch or dinner. Years earlier Bill saved a man's life. George returned the favor, along with a little someone we didn't even know yet.

What do we actually own over an entire life? In a way, everything is rented. Even our children are borrowed for an undisclosed period of time. We care for them, but we do not claim them as a possession. In the end, we have to give it all up. Things have a false way of making you feel immortal. *My* home...*my* husband...*my* kids. These are *mine*. How can anything bad happen? The trick is accepting the impermanence of everything here. But I've never been any good at letting go; it has always felt unnatural.

We moved again. This time just across town, to a house owned by the New Canaan Historical Society. Built in the 1920s, it had serious charm and I was excited to live there. Occasionally we would bump into the family who had purchased The Pines. Each time it seemed I was with Natalie, who helped keep me from crying on the spot. Once in a diner, the wife came in with her daughter, and Natalie grabbed my arm. "They're HERE," she whispered. I turned to look. "What? Who is here?" It was THEM, the house buyers. What should we do? We smiled, said hello, and Natalie got behind my wheelchair and starting pushing full force. Bill was no better, but he pretended to be. He said he was fine, but whenever we visited our friends who still lived on the street, he was sure to go the long way, in order to avoid passing our old address. More than once, I dreamt that we still lived there. Each time it was the same...our family was back in the house, but hiding from the new family. We would be discovered and told to leave. I would then remind them that it really was *our* home—even though I knew it wasn't—and beg them to let us stay. After the dreams, I would wake up heartsick. How could I get it back? It was such unrefined emotion, but, that is the nature of dreams, they go about prodding at the thoughts down under, the things we put away to deal with another day. I was still dealing with the house somewhere in my subconscious, and maybe even in my conscious, because I wanted it back.

It took Natalie going back to help me. She decided one afternoon to knock on the door of our old house. She asked the owner if she could go inside and look around. The man, who was also a father of young girls, knew Natalie and kindly obliged. When she came home she said, "Mom, I went to our old house." I was shocked. Being my firstborn, she has always been sensitive to my emotions. Her eyes filled with tears as she spoke, "It didn't feel like our home anymore." Closure. She hugged me and looked closely to see if my reaction mirrored hers. More than sadness and longing, I felt grateful to the man for allowing her to enter, and to say goodbye once more. She needed to see it, to go inside and remember what it felt like to be there. I was proud of her for knowing what to do. Natalie was brave.

Like Dorothy in the Land of Oz, I wanted to find my way home, except I didn't know where it was any longer. Was it east or west? Was it only in the past? Something slipped away, something I wanted and for a moment was in my grasp. I was searching. It didn't seem that I would get there without some sort of hero's journey, as my therapist Alison reminded me so often. Dorothy could not fast forward to Oz to meet the Wizard. First, she had to face danger, make friends, and become her own hero. Only then did she realize that she possessed the power all along.

A full year after we moved into the yellow house owned by the Historical Society, I sat in the bathroom staring at another positive pregnancy test. It was September 2012, the night of Natalie's first high-school homecoming dance and her friends were at our house, wearing short dresses and high heels and looking gorgeous. There was general excitement in the air, but I was locked behind the door, panicked. Should I scream? Cry? Risk telling an already miserable husband? Once Nat left with her friends, I broke the news. "Bill, I need to tell you something, but please do not be upset." He always hated when I said that. And, to be sure, Bill was shocked, maybe too shocked to be upset.

"Show me the test." He went right out to buy another test so we could be sure. The results were consistent. He shook his head, hugged me, but said very little. A few minutes into his disbelief he asked, "How do you feel?" His concerns always centered around me. "Do you think this will be okay for you?"

I shrugged my shoulders. How could I know? Always somewhat fearful of my post-injury pregnancies, I admitted, "I am scared, Bill. I can only think this will not end well." But he would never say no to life. Despite the precariousness of our situation, Bill was not going to try to sway me one way or another. Like he has done throughout our long relationship, he lets me be me. I can't say I always do the same. This latest pregnancy made me feel as if we were being tested again, and I asked him what he thought.

"I don't think of it that way, Annette. I only know I would not change any aspect of our life if it meant we would not have the girls." But he did not have the worry of a pregnancy. Could I do it? Endure nine months of worry at a time when so many things were uncertain? The miscarriages of 2007, 2008, and 2009 were not at the forefront of my thoughts any longer. I did not miss the sorrow. The raw feelings I had finally compartmentalized soon resurfaced. Our entire household was too fragile to take this on, I thought. It was not a good time to have a baby.

A friend of mine had recently given birth to a delightful baby girl. Whenever I saw them at church, I longed to squeeze those sweet baby cheeks but when she would start to fuss, I was relieved that our kids were past the stage of diapers, nursing, and sleepless nights. That said, if someone were to drop a baby at our door, would we not take it in? The short answer was yes. It wasn't that I did or didn't want a baby. I was 45-years-old and the thought had not seriously crossed my mind in years. My heart said yes.

The three years back in New Canaan were an open wound. What remained of our social life dwindled down to almost nothing. People we thought were friends criticized us for having hosted parties back when life was good—as if to suggest that such events were the reason for our current predicament. Yet our difficulties occurred at the same time as they were happening around the world. Many others shared our plight as the housing market collapsed, banks were in jeopardy, and small proprietary funds got snuffed out. It was a treacherous time to be working for oneself.

We considered and reconsidered this pregnancy. There were health concerns—my injury for one, my advanced maternal age (something they never let you forget)—and, of course, Bill's being out of work and undecided as to what he would do next with the exception of the latest on Netflix. I was not merely conflicted, but in the throes of an emotional and spiritual crisis.

I knew I'd want to speak with a priest, but I also felt the need to consult a group of close girlfriends. First, I went to see Ann, George's wife. They knew how Bill was struggling and would clearly understand the terrible timing of a pregnancy. Ann listened carefully. "What do you want to do?" she asked. I didn't know. You could see by her expression that she felt my pain. She never voiced her own opinion but reminded me that, should I decide to have the baby, I would be strong enough. It may have been rather late in life to realize that friends, true friends, the kind who see you through hard times and even give you the benefit of the doubt, are pure gold. But we had them. Dad told me on more than one occasion that if you have two true friends you are lucky. Two? I remember saying that it didn't seem like much. He smiled at me knowing that someday I would understand exactly what he meant. Our number of friends was not impressive, but the quality was. Another good friend (also named Anne) drove with me up to Yale for medical advice. We spent a good deal of time getting to know each other when a mutual friend was dying. We tried to visit our friend as often as we could. Anne always picked me up, and for hours we sat at the bedside of Patti, a beautiful mother and wife who was wasting away with cancer. When I witnessed the way Anne treated Patti, with such dignity and love, I knew I was blessed to know this person. She was a nurse by trade, but not all nurses know how to make a dying person feel human. Many of our conversations revolved around the why question. Why did Patti get cancer? She worked so hard to make a beautiful life for her family. Anne was Jewish, and I Catholic, but there were many more topics about which we agreed than disagreed. Neither one of us could fathom the reason for our friend's suffering. But knowing the depth of her compassion, I asked if she would come with me as I listened and weighed the options of my pregnancy with a specialist. She was not going to judge me, no matter what my final decision.

The doctor whose job included the termination of unwanted pregnancies was soft spoken, kind and compassionate. I liked her immediately. "Do you remember me?" she asked. I tried to place her, but couldn't. "Well, the last time we met, you were in a bad way. I helped with your miscarriage." Now I knew why I did not remember. She continued, "You were so upset, it was terrible." And here we were again. I thought about how strange life can be. I stared at the posters on her office wall, trying hard not to make eye contact for fear of crying.

She was not trying to persuade me, but helping me to objectively consider the possible complications. "My thinking about this pregnancy," she said, "is that it may be too much for you emotionally and too much for you physically." I completely believed that she was thinking of me. We talked for almost two hours. She wrote down a list of statistics explaining my chances for a good pregnancy and a healthy baby. It was safer for me not to have the baby.

I had asked so many questions but finally I knew that it came down to a single one: "Do you think that *this* is a life?" I asked, gesturing to my belly.

She did not hesitate, "Yes, I think it is a stage of life, just like there are babies, then toddlers, who become teenagers; they are all stages of life." It's not my place to make a moral judgment about how she was able to do her job—how she took life from the womb every day. But I knew that her intention was to help mothers, many of whom, she explained, were in desperate situations. Before I left, I made an appointment to come back in two days.

That night, I had a nightmare. A child called to me from the darkness. Maybe I had addressed the physical and emotional components of the decision, but for me, the spiritual one is the only one. *That* is who I am. I've been that way since the days when I considered God to be my first friend. He may be merciful, but I had already condemned myself. I went to see a priest—two, in fact. Father Ian was my friend and spiritual advisor. We got together regularly for prayer, for confession, and to help increase my faith. There were so many questions since my injury that still plagued me. He believed my thoughts about ending the pregnancy were a temptation and a test. He wanted me to trust God, no matter the outcome. (Trust God? How many times had I put my faith in God? Through all my years in a wheelchair, through each miscarriage...I knew better than to believe that trusting God meant everything would be all right.)

I met with Father Peter at the park near our house. He sat on a bench and I pulled my wheelchair up close enough for him to understand that this was to be a very private conversation. He heard me out and responded, "God loves you, no matter what." Had I forgotten? The judgment would be mine. It made me cry. His words comforted me. Did I know or feel that God loved me, or that I mattered to Him at all? I felt beaten down for so long, and maybe *that* was the temptation—to stop believing in love.

The next day, Bill and I went to the ultrasound appointment we'd set up. Five years earlier, I'd miscarried only six weeks into a pregnancy. The decision had been made by nature. Being that much older now, I wondered if nature might once again intervene. Instead, the ultrasound showed a tiny, pea-sized heartbeat. I looked over at Bill. We cried together, but said nothing. The words did not come, and I looked away. Then Bill said, "I know you, Annette, and you know yourself. It isn't about something being right or wrong. No matter how scared you are, no matter what you go through in the next several months, you'll torture yourself every single day of your life if you don't move forward with this pregnancy." Bill accepts me as I am, and I love him for that. It doesn't matter that I have anxiety, can be overly religious, and can't use my legs. The priest's words came to my mind. God loves me.

"Okay," I said to Bill. "I will take this day by day." And we left, clinging to our hope.

We interviewed several doctors. It was paramount to find one who could work with a patient like me. I know I'm not easy. It's not intentional and it's not to be difficult. It's because of what happened and, to be fair, I am sometimes hypochondriacal. (Although I think I've earned that right.) I'm always checking things online, looking through medical journals, doing exactly what the doctors tell you not to do. The perinatologist, Dr. Stella at Greenwich Hospital *got* me, and agreed that

I could come in once a week to check the baby's heartbeat. If things went wrong, she promised to take me in right away for a D&C. Once we reached the 20-week mark, it wasn't necessary to make the weekly trips. The baby was developing normally. We decided not to do additional tests. At each ultrasound Bill took my hand kissed it and said, "It's all going to be fine, Annette." Secretly, I think he hoped for a boy. After the heartbreak of losing one, he didn't want to say the words out loud. Bill is a man in touch with his feminine side. He is gentle, protective, and fun. The girls remind me that he is way more fun than me every time we get in the car. He allows them to listen to "their" music.

"Dad is cool, Mom, don't you get it?" So this time we laughed when the technician told us it was another girl. What else could it be?

I asked for one more look, "Are you sure it's a girl?"

"I do this every day," he said. "Sometimes, the picture isn't that clear, but in this case, it is definitely, absolutely, and positively a girl."

Georgia Grace was born during a super moon, on Sunday, June 23, 2013. Anne rushed to the hospital as soon as she could, and was the first person besides Bill to see Georgia after she was born. Georgia was tiny in part due to my hyperthyroid, a gift of pregnancy, and a condition called marginal cord insertion of the umbilical cord. When Dr. Stella made the discovery during an ultrasound, she said, "Now, Annette, don't look it up. It is going to be fine." I was tempted to do an online search and learn all about it, but I didn't. I didn't look it up once. At just over 5 pounds, she was light and we would need to keep her body warm, but perfect in every way. We named her Georgia because of George. Bill, the girls and I agreed this was a way to honor their special friendship. Bill says now that it was both George and Georgia who resuscitated him from his zombie-like state. He rocked her to sleep every night, and carried her with him throughout the day like a little football. Her tiny fingers wrapped around his reminded him that life was precious, a gift. It gave him the push he needed to keep going.

My last pregnancy and Georgia changed me. Before Georgia, I would have said that, regardless of circumstances, you must always proceed with a pregnancy. Although my core belief has not changed, my compassion has deepened. Dad's example of unconditional love showed me that I must give the same. Whenever I called dad to discuss the pregnancy, it was hard for me to express how I felt knowing his strong support of life. For him, it was more than being a devout Catholic, this was a black and white issue. When I shared how very afraid I was, he shocked me with his response, "Annette, you already know how I feel, but what you do not know is that no matter what you decide I will always love you. Pray about this. I have no doubt that you and Bill will make a good decision." The support I had at home from Bill, my father, the girls and close friends gave me the strength to fight my daily mental and physical battles for nine months. It was time, and as usual it passed. Dr. Stella was steady throughout. Without all of them, I must acknowledge that Georgia may not be here.

I believe in life—in the womb and after—but I will never judge a person for making a different choice. When I look at Georgia, at her little hands and feet, or her twirling in the yard until she is so dizzy she falls over, I recognize that even on the tough days, I'm overjoyed that we said yes.

The first day we were home with Georgia, Father Ian stopped by. He sat down on the bench in the front yard and said, "See Annette, God is good." It was still incredible that she was here and healthy. I shared with Father that I did not know what to make of the whole experience. I did not understand why this life came to its fullness yet the others did not. As Father Ian spoke, that single thought consumed me. I was dumbfounded that this time things went so well. "It was God," he said.

I shook my head. "Of course, everything is God, you can say that. All I can say is I had one good egg left." He smiled. He often said to me that while I struggled with my faith, he believed it was strong, and as important as thoughts are, actions are of even greater consequence. Knowing times were tough and that Bill was still looking for work, a family from Church wanted to help. Suddenly, my thoughts shifted to the baby's nursery. We could purchase a crib, clothing, and maybe, paint the walls pink?

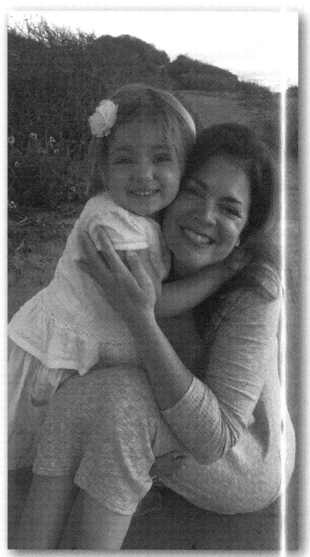

With our Georgia.

I went into the house to tell Bill of our amazing good fortune. He looked at me intently with his green eyes, and responded. "We're moving."

I was stunned. "WHAT? Really?"

"YES," he said. I asked again, and got the same response. I guess the answer was "yes." Before Georgia, we'd wondered where "home" should be and ever since we moved from Hemlock Hill, it was an ongoing conversation. Where was our home? But Georgia's arrival was a game changer for Bill. He wanted to go west. She was also a game changer for me. In Connecticut, we wouldn't be alone in this—we had family, and friends who would visit and help. We discussed it, sort of, made lists of pros and cons, and prayed. But Bill was not staying. He was done with feeling downtrodden, physically, he'd begun to deteriorate. For the sake of his health, both mental and physical, he wanted to go back to California. This time for him. Georgia's birth gave him a single moment of clarity and, with that, he wanted to act. How could I refuse? The man who'd carried me up the stairs for months because I viewed the purchase of a stair climber as a defeat deserved the same allegiance in return. A healthy baby was a blessing, this was a new start. I tried to convince myself I could do it.

Before we made a final decision, I confided in several friends. On a walk with the baby one afternoon, my friend Kathy listened to our plans and said, "My only concern is that once you get there, it will be just the two of you, all alone, and you might need more than that. It won't be good for it to be just you and Bill against the world."

"Yes," I agreed, "that scares me too." Although my reservations were not addressed, we left quickly. As we pulled away from our street, I realized we had not even said goodbye to some of our closest friends. We simply appeared to vanish. It was a bold move, any way you look at it, maybe even a foolish one. It did not feel like a beginning, but the end.

The one comfort I had in our move back was knowing that my Uncle Jim, Dad's brother, would be near. He lived in Los Angeles. It was more than 100 miles from San Diego, but still. Two of Uncle Jim's daughters also lived close by, so we would have loving people, family, with whom to share holidays and special occasions. Less so, the joys of day-to-day interactions, but it was something.

Uncle Jim was a special person in my life since I first became a Fenwick. He is very much like my father (so easy to love), and also very much his own man. While Dad never had a career that fully manifested his talents and passions, Uncle Jim was born with a gift for mathematics, which he put to practical use as an engineer. He is endlessly fascinating to talk with about every imaginable subject because he actually knows something about nearly everything. One afternoon, while we sat on the shores of the beach, he used math to explain the vibrations that ocean waves make as they break on the shore. My mind doesn't easily grasp such concepts, but he's a patient teacher. When his formulas get ahead of my intellect, we can easily switch to conversations about the existence of God. Like my father, his faith is childlike, and for such an intellectual I've often wondered why it was so easy for him not to need to know everything. You can prove theories with math, but you can never "prove" God. Some things are left to faith and to humility. Uncle Jim has an abundance of both.

At the rehearsal dinner the night before our wedding, Uncle Jim stood up to toast Bill and me. Afterward, Aunt Barb (his wife) confided that such a public expression of emotions and love wasn't something Uncle Jim did easily. But we meant that much to him.

Although we never discussed it, I think that Uncle Jim sees in Bill and me the same deeply held love that he always felt for Aunt Barb. His devotion to her throughout their married life was a testament to what it means to love your spouse. Although she died several years ago, he includes her in every conversation. When we visit him, he'll look at her picture and say, "Isn't she just beautiful. I sure was lucky." And he was. I cherish him.

The home we had arranged to move into once we arrived in San Diego turned out to be less than wheelchair accessible. It was my fault. I had only seen pictures of the house online, and it reminded me of "home" with its white kitchen and wood floors. From the photos, we could see there was a step that divided the first floor, but it was only ten inches so we assumed it could be ramped. On its own, that was not enough to cause us to look elsewhere, but once we saw the yard and the location set near the top of a very steep hill, we realized there were too many obstacles for me with my chair and an infant. It would make going outside with Georgia (once she could walk) very difficult and perhaps even dangerous to navigate. The yard was filled in with a substance similar to gravel that was not conducive to moving smoothly with a wheelchair.

Uncle Jim offered to let us regroup at his home. It was important to find a house quickly, but I was in need of rest. Whenever we stayed with him, he pampered us. Each morning, he made the girls poached eggs every bit as perfect as Julia Child's. He made sure we were all comfortable, giving Bill, Georgia and me the first-floor master bedroom, and finding space for the older girls with his blow up mattresses. We felt safe with him, and there was a part of me that did not want to leave. Our new life felt so unsettled, and his home held within it the memories of a full life, one of love, family, and adventure. With school about to begin, we had to get organized. We found a home that was within walking distance of the public grade school, perfect for Ingrid and Mia, and jumped on it. The physical act of moving our things from one place to another always depressed me. To lighten the load before we left Connecticut, we had to give away—and basically ditch—a lot of our belongings. Lawn furniture, work-out equipment, even a kayak that Bill got me for my birthday. (Kayaking was a sport we'd hoped to do more often together, but it would have to wait.)

One item we kept was the piano, but just barely. It's such a part of my history, and a connection to Connie, to leave it behind would have been like giving away a part of myself. I'd learned to play when I was little. Mom and Dad purchased sheet music to their favorite songs, and I would perform nightly concerts in our family room. Having developed a keen appreciation of the Tommy Dorsey Orchestra, I chose "I'll Be Seeing You" as my special dance with Dad on our wedding day. Days after I was hurt, as I lay in the hospital bed, still in shock thinking about what was lost, I realized I might never play the piano again. I had my hands, true, but the foot pedals add a depth to the sound. For a few years, I played with no pedal. Eventually, intense rehab helped my right foot become strong enough to press down. Lifting up the foot was a weaker motion, but good enough to allow me to feel in command. After playing for any length of time, my foot went into spasm, but for only a few minutes. The girls do not yet share my love of classical music, nor does Bill—hence the long-ago night of Beethoven's Seventh. But knowing my passion for Bach and Beethoven, Bill once purchased a series of concert tickets to the New York Philharmonic. He surprised me on Christmas Eve, 1999, with a box containing tickets for the following spring. We never got to go.

As much as I resisted, things became so difficult after the move that I had to sell some personal items, presents given to me by Bill in better times. They were just "things," I realized, but they had sentimental value, and I knew with each sale that they would be gone forever. "Is this what you want me to do?" I kept asking Bill.

His pained response: "It is ultimately up to you." He just wanted to get it over with. Georgia accompanied us on one visit to the pawn shop to sell jewelry and silverware. The actual storefront had bars across the windows. It felt like a prison, with doors that had to be unlocked to enter and to exit. They even employed guards. The people coming in and out looked strung out on drugs and, like us, desperate. It was not the ideal place for a six-month-old, but the gentle weight of her little body in my lap kept me from becoming unhinged. The man who owned the shop had sensitive eyes. He looked at Georgia and then at me. "I know you're upset to be here," he said. "But *she* is your real treasure." His words consoled me. This was distressing but I had the items to sell. With one squeeze of my chubby baby girl, I let go of my possessions I'd gotten joy from all of them—our house, the pretty furniture, the furnishings we'd so happily amassed. In my "fairy tale" life, I'd envisioned passing them down to our daughters. In a way, I did pass them on, only to recipients unknown, and I hoped they would find pleasure in them. As for my precious Georgia, her life could not be weighed and measured.

It was difficult for me to move from house to house with teens, pre-teens, and a baby. But what was it like for the girls?

When we first moved back to Connecticut in 2010, Natalie reconnected with some good friends, but things quickly changed once she entered the high school. She did not have a productive freshman year. I couldn't figure it out. She was bright, pretty, fun, and also a talented athlete. After she'd attended weeks of lacrosse practice, when I asked the coach about an upcoming game, she turned to me with a blank face. "Your daughter has not been at one practice." Stunned, I didn't know what to say. Bill had mentioned more than once that she never looked sweaty when he'd picked her up at the school. Where had she been going? What had she been doing? Not understanding what was at play in her reckless behavior, I blamed myself and our situation.

Unintentionally, I think I put pressure on Natalie. She was the only one of our children to play a part in Act One of "The Dream" I had so desperately wanted to fulfill. She may have known this without my saying so and put too much pressure on herself. Whenever she made a mistake, I took it as a personal failure. To hold on to the dream, I was determined to ensure her success. It was hard for me to understand her and, as she said so often, "Mom, you want me to be *you*, and I'm not!" After hearing that so many times, one night I asked myself, "Do I want her to be me?" No, I wanted her to be the *me* I never was. When I looked at her, I knew she had what it took to pull it off. It was not fair, and thankfully she was strong enough to rebuff me when I overwhelmed her. The girls will each have their unique dreams, and they need not be clouded by my unfulfilled hopes. They are not me or Bill and can't finish off our story line.

Our decisions for ourselves and the girls were being made from a place of pain and suffering. Each poor decision led to others. One was the lawsuit: in the end, we accepted a settlement instead of going to trial because we longed for it to finally be over. I wanted to pay off the house. Bill wanted to fund the business. Neither choice was bad. He understood my desire to know that the house was safely ours, yet we chose to bolster the business. I felt guilty about all Bill had done for me, knowing he'd sacrificed his work. He was frustrated that the lawyers never once considered that he was an entrepreneur, working on his own while caring for me around the clock. Anger and guilt, it was through the lens of these emotions that we decided everything. It became a vicious cycle of regret.

Somewhere during our time in the desert (literally and figuratively), we stopped having fun. Life became monotonous and dull for all of us, each in different ways. We were not moving forward (or backward). We were stagnant, and stagnation leads to death. The pressure of our decisions began to weigh heavily on us. No one deserved to be at the center of our family arguments, but everyone had a turn. Bill and I both wanted to give the girls a childhood comparable to his own, but one with the religious foundation that meant so much to me. But we were not succeeding on either front. Every day felt like the day before. None of us had any gas in the tank; we were just there, together in the house, trying not to throw plates. Little things caused the girls to argue, a lost shoe, a borrowed article of clothing, or whoever finished the ice cream while everyone else was sleeping. It troubled me to see them like this, and I played peacemaker reminding them to be nice, that change disorients everyone, and we needed to have patience with ourselves and each other. From 2009 to 2015, we moved five times. I could not find the simple things to make a house feel like a home.

Christmas was the most difficult. Once I unpacked the worn boxes of decorations there was always something missing or in pieces. It was hard for me to be lighthearted about it, but I tried because I knew the girls were closely watching my every expression just waiting to see how I would react. They still wanted Christmas to be special and they were waiting, waiting for us to find our motivation. Waiting for the usual traditions to return, like the train set under the tree. But we could not find it within ourselves to hide our frustration, and we never did find the train set.

On my worst days, I dread the conversations we are likely to have with the girls once they've grown, had time to reflect on their childhood, and share their opinions about the rocky road we've all traveled. (They don't hold back now!) Bill and I will need to be strong enough—and humble enough—to accept how they eventually make sense of it all.

How was it that we arrived to this point? Together, Bill and I have compiled a list of regrets, and periodically debated the events that changed our once-sweet life.

"If only we'd paid off the house right away, we would have a home now," I blurt out.

He responds with, "I wanted to move long before you could get around to the idea." That was true.

"Okay," I counter, "maybe we shouldn't have left Chicago."

"Maybe we should have stayed in Bermuda," he retorts.

And Bill's undeniable truth: "I always told you that the house was an investment. But having you pursue walking was more important."

"Yes," I agree. And with those words, the guilt begins to pile up again. "Bill, you've done so much for me. I don't believe anything is your fault. I only wanted to save the house." There it was, my truth, the house was something I wanted. It was safe there. I was Holly Golightly in *Breakfast at Tiffany's* a scared girl in search of a place where nothing bad would happen.

Bill felt strongly that any magic he'd once had disappeared the day I came home in a wheelchair. This is why he eventually insisted that we had to make a change. Early on, we worked as a team to battle the reality of my injury. The girls, too. We all gave up things we wanted for the dream of me walking again. For months, Bill carried me upstairs to bed every night because he understood that I wasn't ready to face certain inevitabilities. There was an adjustment period, and mine was long. He never wanted me to give up the fight, so long as I wanted to continue. Eventually, though—and before I was ready—he felt the need to try something new. It didn't mean I had to give up therapy. He just instinctively felt that things would never be the same for us in New Canaan.

One of Bill's best friends from high school lost her husband on September 11th. Meredith and Pete had two gorgeous blond haired daughters — one was the same age as Natalie. Before we were married, we visited New Canaan, and attended a party they hosted. It was Christmastime, and the house was aglow. The lit fires, candlelight, and freshly shucked oysters made such an impression on me. Afterward I said to Bill, "I can see us living here." They were an exceptional family, and when we moved into town our friendship deepened. But soon after the tragedy she left Connecticut. Years later, as we struggled to define home, Bill said to me, "That's what *we* should have done." I hadn't understood what he meant. It always surprised me that Meredith left, but I understand now. I was unable to embrace a new dream. Too afraid, or maybe I lacked the creativity. I can only remember us having versions of the same conversation many times before I really heard him.

The day before Mother's Day 2014, I fell out of my wheelchair and broke my femur. We were back in San Diego for one year and were already inspecting the latest list of houses on the rental market because the owners of our current home were returning from China. As we rushed from one vacant house to the next, I became agitated. They all looked the same, and I couldn't picture us living in any of them. I still did not grasp that parts of my life were gone for good. As we exited the final house of the day, I moved too quickly and my wheels got stuck in the door jam.

Before I had time to call out, "Bill," I landed on the concrete. The x-rays confirmed that the break was right above the knee joint. I asked for pain meds right away. The sensation in my legs made a much better comeback than my motor function, but pain often registered as either too strong or too weak and, where I once resisted taking any medications, I learned to appreciate what they can do for you. After gathering a few opinions from the orthopedic surgeons (my least favorite specialty), they decided that my bones were not strong enough for surgery. The pins might not hold, and there was the risk of infection. Although surgery would have made for a shorter recovery, the decision was made to avoid potential complications by setting my leg—ouch!—and placing a fiberglass cast from the top of my left thigh straight down to my stubby toes.

(The last time I had broken a bone, it had been my ankle. Then, the doctor looked at me and asked what I wanted him to do? "Well," I said, exasperated, "what do you normally do?" He said, "I'd put on a boot or cast it, but you're not walking, so I suppose it doesn't really matter." We left his office and found a new orthopedist. Clearly, there was nothing I could have said to get him to care about me. I once wrote an essay about hope and medicine that briefly addressed the doctor-patient relationship. Waiting in the lobby of a doctor's office gives you time to think. What did I want from my doctors? I recalled a passage from Genesis where Jacob wrestles with God. "I won't let you go until you bless me," Jacob says. Even the doctors who we decided were not going to be part of the team mattered to me, and I wanted their blessing.)

It was going to be a long, hot summer. Back to being dependent on Bill for every bathroom visit, and there were plenty, day and night. Georgia was not even a year old and didn't sleep well. Natalie continued to give us trouble with school. She had a dismal performance during her sophomore year. We appealed to the Catholic high school. It was late to accept her, but they said yes, and we hoped that her junior year would be a fresh start. But it wasn't just Natalie; none of the girls were equipped to help me while I was laid up. They all had growing pains of their own. Bill carried the brunt of it all. For as much as a new injury brought back the memory of my first days in captivity, I barely realized how much they affected Bill, until one night I woke to find him pacing the room.

He stood in the dark in his t-shirt and boxers. It was 2 a.m. It was unclear how long he was up, but I don't think he ever went to bed.

"What's going on?" I asked him.

"The day you lost your legs was the day I lost everything. It wasn't just *you*. Do you understand that?"

Where was this coming from, I wondered, and why now? "Yes, I do," I whispered, as he continued his rant.

"I lost track of my life, my work. Everything became about caring for you. I don't even know who I am anymore!" He started yelling, waking up the house. I began to cry.

"Why are *you* crying?" he screamed. "*I'm* the one who should be crying. What am I going to do now? How do I rebuild a career at my age? I'm alone. We're alone. We are done, and I may as well disappear."

"Please, Bill, don't do that. These girls are counting on us to make things right. Not a perfect life, but to be there."

He calmed somewhat, but said, "Annette, you do not understand me. You never have. The pressure I feel to get our life back on track and to take care of you and the girls is insurmountable."

"Who helped you with Georgia?" He pointed at our baby, asleep on the bed. "Who held her and walked her all the nights you did not?"

It was true. The pregnancy was mine, but that first year of late nights was largely Bill's. I nursed her, but he held and walked her when she was fussy, irritable, or had a fever from shots the day before. He carried a large part of the load when Georgia was born, every bit as much as me. Would it have helped to put some sort of context around what he was feeling? To mention that the girls were healthy? That we still had each other? I stayed awake with him, but kept quiet. I never want to see Bill upset. He's a good man with a good heart. And I get that the pressure builds up over time. He saw the look of guilt on my face, and said, "Annette, I'm sorry. You're my wife. I am so glad you're here. We were meant to help each other through this life." He had said things like this before, that I'd saved him from his demons when he was young, and that he knew with absolute certainty I was the one for him. It happened on the golf course in Bermuda, he said he was standing over a putt on the seventh hole and thought of us walking along Fullerton Avenue in Chicago. A feeling of peace washed over him and he decided right then that I was even more important than whether or not he made the putt...a pretty big revelation. But, to hear him tell the story convinced me that his love was true. He believed we were destined to be one. It was terrifying to think that the pressure we were under was great enough to compromise that. It confused us, and made us forget, at least momentarily, what we mean to each other.

He eventually fell asleep, but now I lay awake. I flipped through the channels on the television, trying to find a film to distract me. Had I asked too much of him? Would we be able to stay married, and happily? My leg was throbbing inside the cast, and the bitterness threatened to swallow me up. Then we will have truly lost, I thought to myself.

Hearing the distress in Bill's voice made me wish I never survived my initial injury. The entire broken leg drama brought my anguish back to its infancy, and I wondered if I had really forgiven anyone. Or maybe it was something that I'd have to do again and again? The anesthesiologist who gave me the epidural came freshly into my mind. There she was, her uncombed blond hair, red face, and hot tears, standing at the end of my hospital bed. This time I wanted to yell at her, "Guess what? I'm going to have problems FOR THE REST OF MY LIFE." The time to scream had long passed. My thoughts turned raw and ugly. Decisions we made during the lawsuit haunted me. Maybe Bill was right, we should have fought for more. If my bones were going to crumble every time I moved, I wanted security. (I also wanted a flat in Paris with a crystal chandelier in the bathroom.) I had friends who'd endured months lying on their stomachs while a pressure wound healed. And more than one had chosen to take their own lives as the relentlessness of their situations wore them down. I knew I was being ridiculous. The only question was where I would find the reserve of strength necessary to keep going? It took one fall for me to regress into painful, discarded and forgotten feelings.

Only two weeks after my cast was removed, the moving truck arrived. I loved that our new house had pretty wooden floors upstairs, but needed to stop caring about the rest of it. Thoughts of trying to recreate our dream home had not served me well. We had a roof over our children's heads. That was something to be thankful for.

"God, help me to do right by these girls. I love them. Help me to love them more." That's my first prayer after communion. God had trusted me to mother them even with a spinal cord injury. I just didn't always know how. These past few years since moving back to San Diego have been the most difficult for me; they've required something that I did not have, or if I did, I didn't have enough of it. It was essential that Bill focus on work, something he'd needed to do for a long time. To honor that commitment, I needed to change. When he is gone at his new job and the girls have left for school, the house feels like a stranger. Only Georgia reminds me of who I am. She draws my attention away from the frustration of leftover pieces of furniture that have no purpose. I have not been able to give her the things I gave the other girls. She does not seem to mind.

Although we'd moved only a few miles, we would be living in a different school district. It didn't matter that the school year had already begun—in the State of California, when you move from one district to another, you're required to change schools. Fortunately, because Natalie and Anna were in the Catholic school, which didn't have such stringent geographic regulations, they would remain unaffected by our move. But Ingrid and Mia, who were both happy at their current grade school, were slated to be transferred. It stressed me to think about what was in store for them. As much as Bill and I tried, we could not shield our girls from everything, but it was important to initiate an appeal process on the behalf of our two younger ones. Because Ingrid was in sixth grade (her final year in that school), the district made the allowance, and gave her little sister a grace year. But they cautioned that, should we not move back into the district, Mia would have to attend a new school the following year. I worried about how well the girls were coping with so much change. My friend Claire once counseled me, "Annette, if you can be happy, the girls will follow your lead."

I was sincerely trying to be positive, but the remnants of our former life infiltrated my spirit. Once you let everything go, what do you do? Growing up, I remember a friend's mother telling me, "It doesn't matter the size of your home, just keep it clean. There are no messes in Heaven." So, as I cleaned up each day after Bill and the girls had left for work and school, I prayed. And I began to feel that, although mine was a small life, I had a role to play. "God, let me serve my family." Wasn't that what I'd always asked for in my prayers? The time in daily prayer was good, and allowed me to feel that, housebound though I was for most of the day, I was putting some love out there.

Once the school logistics were set, I started to assess those pieces of furniture we'd decide to bring west with us. They were looking shabby and, like us, weren't getting any younger. I found that I felt more control over our living situation when I could fill in the cracks, clean, or paint our belongings. Georgia tried to help me, in her way. She drew on the furniture, ate the dog's food, and tried to catch bees in the backyard. But that's an 18-month-old for you.

I went online to see what I could reasonably accomplish. Turns out Palmolive and a scrub brush really will clean a couch! I had never refinished anything, but was willing to try. So I bought some sandpaper and got to work on our coffee table. With a bucket of white paint and a helping hand from Annie, (one of my three friends in San Diego), it looked almost new. I thought that, if I could do these things—if I could keep life going—then we, as a family, would have something left to fight for.

When I see a homeless person walking along the road with a packed shopping cart, I wonder three things: What happened to them? Can I do anything to help? And, what is in the cart?

I know now what happens. It takes a little bit of bad luck, one or two poorly made decisions, and no one left to help. There you are. The reason I was adamant about things staying "put together" was because I pictured us as a family with our last Lego and broken TV remote wondering what happened.

We came out to San Diego on our own and, with the exception of Uncle Jim and his family, we have been alone. I often say to Bill, "If we left here tomorrow no one would even notice." He denies it, but it is nonetheless true. Is it ever too late to realize what your friends mean to you? Now that we have lived here for nearly three years I think I know. We are not meant to be separated from others or live in isolation, although I have found the phrase from Dr. Seuss's *Oh the Places You'll Go* to be true: "Whether you like it or not, alone is something you'll be quite a lot!"

Before I became disabled, when people shared with me their need to "do it alone," it always left me cold. Those who understand just how much we need one another are usually the first to offer their help to others. I experienced that firsthand during my month at Yale-New Haven Hospital. It wasn't for the sake of rewards, but because they knew the greater purpose of being there. I feel that absence of help now. It is like a gaping hole in the fabric of my life. We were a family in need. And it doesn't take a disability to make you vulnerable. It could be losing a job. It could be poverty. It could be grief. It's easier—or at least more comfortable—to turn a blind eye to those in need. But, our girls, who have very personally witnessed the effects of kindness and generosity, know the difference it has made to us; and that when we were down, that was all we had. They are young, and too often engrossed in their iPhones, but still impressionable. I hope that they notice what is happening around them, that they're inspired to act with compassion, and that they never forget the hands that reached out for ours when we had nothing to hold onto.

As I struggled to find the proper end for our story, my Dad beckoned. He had endured heart attacks, diabetes, even a small stroke, and his body was fragile. My own anxieties had me questioning whether I could handle the trip and, clearly, we could not afford for all of us to fly to Chicago. In the end, Natalie, Anna, and I went. It was my first flight (ever) without Bill. Natalie was 17 and

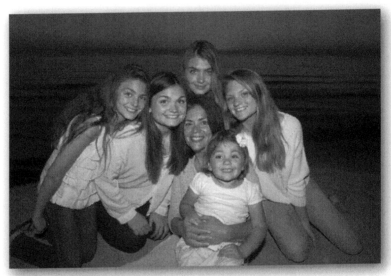

All our girls.

Anna 15, old enough now to give me any emotional and physical support I might need.

Our trip coincided with my 30th high-school reunion. Another source of anxiety. In the end, I savored every moment of it. My friends—many of whom I hadn't seen in years--still saw me in the way I wished to be seen and maybe once was. One of my favorite teachers, Mrs. Paulson, was there. She's had a special ability to communicate how deeply she cared for her students. During the reunion, she leaned in close and said, "I remember you, Annette. You stood in front of my desk explaining some discovery to me with so much passion. After you left, I thought to myself, she is going to be something." What a lovely thing to hear. To be thought of in this way moved me so. I still wished to be that young, enthusiastic girl. That night, I felt like the homecoming queen.

My Dad was my first love on this earth, yet I had not seen him in nearly six years. I could barely contain my joy when I arrived at his apartment. We hugged for a long time. He looked older (we both did). He moved slowly, with the help of a walker, but had dressed up for our visit and was as sharp as ever. We sat around a little table where my brother Tom arranged snacks for us. We made small talk to start—yes, the flight was fine; the family back home was good, healthy; and Georgia (who he'd never met) was finally talking. His place was small, and filled with odd pieces of furniture, some worn out, some antique; Dad did not care a bit. He was happy to sit at his kitchen table and look out the window, which overlooked a meadow. He could name nearly every species of bird that came to visit. I told him about the reunion, what a wonderful night it had been, and Mrs. Paulson's parting words. He smiled so tenderly. "Oh, Annette, I remember her!"

"Dad, she was so wrong. I am a colossal failure. Things have not worked out for us. I have not risen to the circumstances set before me. To say that I tried is not good enough."

"But, it *is* good enough, Annette. You are my daughter and I love you. That makes you someone." What else could I want or need? I had his stamp of approval forever. He asked that I sit alone with him, just the two of us.

"Dad, before you say what you want to say, can I ask you something?"

"Of course," he said.

"Do you ever regret anything?" I wanted to know.

"What would I regret?" he asked.

"I don't know, but maybe wish your life was different?"

"No," he said. "Not at all. I am happy, and more than that, I am content." He continued, "I want to read something to you. He pulled a small prayer card from his pocket. "I say this prayer for Bill every day, multiple times a day. He will find work again,

Annette, and I know the job that he should have—one with a future, one with benefits [that's a Dad for you], and one where he works away from home, so as not to be distracted. [He found the exact one only two months later.] Don't worry, Annette. Pray this prayer with me. We are strong if we do it together."

"Yes, of course, Dad, I will pray with you."

Take my hand O Blessed Mother
Hold me firmly lest I fall
I grow nervous while moving around and humbly on thee call
Guide me over every crossing
Watch me when I am on the stairs
Let me know that you're beside me
Listen to my fervent prayers.
Bring me to my destination safely along the way
Bless my every undertaking
And my duties for the day
And when the evening creeps upon me
I'll never fear to be alone
Once again O Blessed Mother
Take my hand and lead me home. Amen

Later, we went to his room. Pictures of Mom covered the walls. She was so pretty. He said that he still talked to her every day and felt that she was with him in a way he could not fully explain. It comforted me to hear that. He assured me that he wasn't lonely, that each day he enjoyed his prayer time, his quiet, and his view from the kitchen table. For most of my life, I've worried that Dad would depart from us too soon, and then I realized that no matter when it happened, it would be too soon. His complete acceptance of me is unmatched by anyone, and *that* is what defines a father to me. He has been my constant cheerleader, whether it was for a good grade, a good deed, or just listening to me play the piano. In his mind, things are never as grim as what I might present, even when I've adopted Eeyore's gloom-and-doom attitude.

Being in Chicago again flooded my heart with delightful memories. I took the girls to Bill's and my favorite pizzeria and we walked the old neighborhood. We photographed the sidewalk where he and I had engraved our names in front of the three-story walk up twenty years earlier. We stopped at St. Clements Church and the girls patiently listened as I retold the story of my walk up the aisle, holding tightly to my Dad while making my way toward Bill. "Don't cry, Mom." I asked that they join me in prayer before the statue of the Blessed Mother. On our way out, there happened to be a bride making her way up the church steps. I knew it would embarrass the girls if I spoke to her, so I whispered, "Dearest God, bless her on this special day. Let her life be full of joy, and many years with her love. Protect them from harm. Let it not go badly." Just as the priest had described on the day of our union, we are flying through the clouds with no instruments—only faith, hope, and love. I felt Natalie's hand on my shoulder. "Come on, Mom, it's time to go." She called me away from the memory and we left.

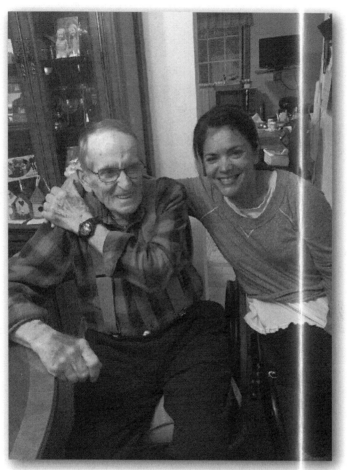

With Dad on our last visit. (2016)

As our plane took off from Chicago, I had one of the girls close the window shade so that I could pretend none of it was happening. I'd found the courage to be there for my Dad, and my love was greater than my fear. My daughters helped me find the strength to be there. It was real life, not the fairy tale. It was another bride's turn, with me in a wheelchair, my daughters growing up, and my Dad nearing his eternal reward. Where did it leave us? I peeked out the window, but couldn't see the city beneath us, and I sighed with relief. We headed toward the sunset.

Weeks after the reunion, I heard from a friend who wrote to say that she wished we'd connected at the party, and that she was still thinking about me. I responded immediately telling her how much I'd enjoyed the reunion and asked about her life. She told me that her husband had committed suicide a few years earlier, and that hers had been a road of anger, forgiveness, and starting over. They'd had money problems, which he'd kept from her. She disclosed that she'd lost everything, was living with her parents now, and only wished that her husband had shared his burden with her because having him in her life was more important than their home or possessions.

As I read her words, I was stunned over her tragic loss, and also ashamed. We began a lengthy conversation about regret, and sorrow, when it can't be changed and what we do with it. I explained that Bill was lost for a period of time, his business had collapsed, and that his wellbeing was of great concern to all who loved him. For years he'd walked a thin rope, and our family was in danger of losing so much more than my idea of home.

This woman and I shared an incredible moment of revelation, our wounds exposed across the miles, and I could not help but wonder if the conversation was more than coincidence. There have been long periods where I experience darkness, where the drama of life plays out in ways that seem to disprove the existence of God, and then, with her correspondence, came a ray of light. I smiled at the thought that God had put us together. It seemed I needed to hear her story in order to reach a deeper understanding of my own. For as much as that is possible for any of us to lift the burdens for another, I wanted to lessen hers. But she had lessened mine. What would have happened had I lost Bill—an infinitely greater loss than my legs, a house, and pure devastation for the girls, a loss from which they would never fully recover. Bill is with us, thank God, ever present for soccer games and family dinners. For the girls and for me. It matters little if the table we sit at is old or new.

Yes, disability defines you. But it has also added another color to my palette and, should I use it well, I still have time to make something beautiful. Again, I thought of Paul, the tent maker. "*I am not saying this because I am in need, for I have learned to be content, whatever the circumstances. I know what it is to be in need, and I know what it is to have plenty. I have learned the secret of being content in any and every situation, whether well fed or hungry, whether living in plenty or in want. I can do all this through Him who gives me strength."*

My Dad wasn't able to provide extravagances for us. He couldn't afford to pay for college, or our wedding. But, he gave me something irreplaceable: the belief that I possessed intrinsic worth. I do not know how he did it. But it is why I chose such a fine person to marry. I believed I was worth being loved. Dad reminded me that we are all works in progress, we do not achieve perfection, and should we think we have "arrived", we have lost humility. My not wanting to disappoint him is the reason I have not thrown in the towel after hitting the curb so many times. I still want him to be proud of the woman I strive to be, even given my weaknesses. A veil parted when my old friend shared her experience with me. Nothing I lost matters to me as much as Bill does.

~

Today

BILL LIVES WITH SUCH PASSION and zest, but together we share a damaged space. It may be because we were both, in a sense, "orphaned," not literally, but figuratively, and then together we found home. It goes well beyond friendship, passion, or vows; maybe he is where I found God. But given that there was little to believe in, that the world became an undistinguishable color after my injury, my faith stemmed from us. God did not forget me completely, Bill was my reminder. He left me with a person to share the indescribable joy and the unrelenting sorrow.

To say that we've made it this far entirely alone would be untrue. When we both reached a point where we turned to one another and neither had any more to give, family and friends were there. Uncle Jim said that when you attend a couple's wedding, you commit to helping them see their promise to fruition. It was also through the gift of others that we were able to keep our promise.

Friends of mine have shared with me that they believe they are better people for their injuries. I think they believe that because, in order to go on, they must. We cannot change the past, but if it were possible, I would. I recognize that one change can be the catalyst for many more. Shortly before my injury, I'd received my letter of acceptance to the Master of Divinity program at Yale. How would our life have changed down that path? Would we have had more children? Would I have been career oriented and not family centered? Would Bill and I have remained so close? But there is the downside to consider. Had this not happened, would we have lost our home? Would our friendships have flourished instead of diminished? Would our family relationships have remained intact? And, come apart they did, mostly because of money. Shakespeare wrote, "Neither a borrower nor a lender be." I don't necessarily agree with this—because I don't know if it's possible to *not be* one or the other—but will say that we've experienced generosity beyond our wildest expectations. And we've felt the exact opposite—punished, demoralized, and degraded.

On our first wedding anniversary, Bill came up with the idea to have us pose for a picture every year on that date, no matter where we were. He wanted to document us growing old together. We look so young, so sweet in that first photo. Now, when I have the mental strength to open the box that holds the record of our years together, I notice the subtle changes, and my heart is filled with overwhelming sadness. There's a poignant quote in Dietrich Bonhoeffer's *Letters & Papers from Prison:* "time is the most valuable thing that we have, because it is the most irrevocable."

Is home a beginning or an end? What makes any place home? The people? The memories? Or, is home something familiar to us, like the smell of turkey on a Thanksgiving morning. Home for me has always meant a going back instead of forward. It is shrouded in the memories I choose to hold on to. One night as Mia and I snuggled in bed to watch "Once Upon A Time," the character of Rumpelstiltskin said, "If you spend all of your time in the past, you can never build your future." I thought about that—the past can be a trap, where time does not stand still but evaporates. Should your past be something wonderful, it's tantalizing to stay there. The vision of a future "forever" home eludes me, and the physical structure we call home right now feels like a place where we store our stuff instead of one where we create new memories. Our recent dwellings have become a series of lonely addresses that represent transition and upheaval. It seems I am somewhat lost.

What remains is the metaphor of *home*, which is full of distinct moments that remind me of who I am. It is that which comforts me. Sometimes it's a pumpkin sitting on a lonely porch. Or the way a curtain sways in the breeze of an open window. Often it is a particular fragrance wafting through the air that brings me back. These small events connect me to something familiar and evoke a sense of my being a part of something more; something mystical. So the questions linger: Is home fragments of what once was? A dream of what I hope will be? Or what actually is? Maybe it doesn't matter. Yet each time we pile into the car headed to another destination, I feel that I am floating in the air with no direction and no purpose. Home provides an anchor. Without it, I am adrift. This may not be something that everyone needs; I only recognize what it does for me. It is no coincidence that I had my longest run with the fewest anxiety attacks when we lived on Hemlock Hill. Not right away because so much happened, but once life had a rhythm and it felt like it was ours, that void did not enter as frequently. There were probably many factors that played a role—my parents were there, our neighbors were like family, I saw Alison every week, and most of all, Bill. He was with me all of the time. When I reflect on why, through such turmoil, my anxiety was relatively dormant, I must look past the house, and to him. Is it a terrible thing if a person has that effect on you? Not for me, but maybe for him.

When I met Bill, there was no doubt we would bind our two lives to live as one. We were meant to be, home was our being together, and anything else was vanity. For the first time, I felt

I belonged somewhere, not out of duty or obligation, but out of pure, unblemished love. I did not need to convince him that I was worthy, and the simplicity of his affection meant we could define our home wherever we were. Bill has always been my greatest joy and deepest consolation. Our home never seemed to be only a place when we began. But, while love may have been enough to satisfy us, love creates, and new life emerged from our life. When confronted with the needs of young children, another definition of "home" became necessary. Home took on multiple meanings and became an opportunity to create something new as well as make right the shortcomings of childhood. I did not want to be my Mom. My children were my opportunity to do better.

To this day, after twenty years together and all that's happened, whenever Bill enters the room, my heart jumps. He is the one person I wish to spend every day with and have next to me at night. He is the best part of my life, even now. Especially now. Bill remains my one true love. He was the impetus for my fairy tale, even before I knew him. He was my prime force, the mover in my life whose love gave me the courage to try to make even the most outlandish dream a reality. And, to my astonishment, I realize that, although imagination can take us far, reality is far superior to anything I could have imagined. In the world you create in make believe, you never make a wrong step. Life guarantees nothing will go as planned, or it may even go tragically wrong. When presented with the pain that is the inevitable result of actual love, we recoil or regret. I often ask people who've spent ample time on this planet the same question I posed of

Dad, "What would I do differently?" He'd said, "What could I have done?" My answer might be to become the daughter my father always believed in, only sooner. He certainly gave me a fine example. However given the disappointments and sufferings, there is only one thing I can say I am certain I would not change. I would marry Bill again without pause. His presence by my side, whether in a hospital room, or our bedroom, made agony not just endurable, but beautiful. He lit a path in my darkness, which allowed me to find the road back. He cared enough about who I was to not allow me to let her go. He took on the full weight of my burdens, and was not rewarded, but misunderstood. While I found my way, he lost his. It may even be true that he gave his life for mine; the ultimate act of heroism. God being good offered me the occasion to save him and, to the best of my ability, I tried to return his uncompromising devotion. Symbolic as it was to blow out our individual candles in order to light one together, we have become one in what we have given to each other.

Deacon John moved to Indiana several years after my injury. Before he left, he sent me a card with the inscription, "grow where you are planted." Being adopted, I craved roots. Instead, the opposite of what I thought I needed to thrive happened. I have been planted and transplanted. There is no place to call home, it exists as a fantasy of what was and will now never be. Our home remains transient, but is more than hazily defined by us together, no matter the numbers that make up our address. It is here we stumble and fall, keep each other going, experience joy, and struggle to make meaning. I am still like a child groping in the darkness,

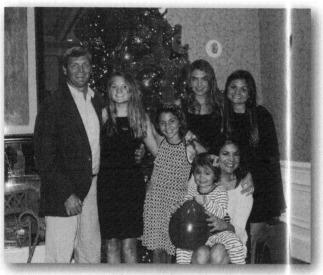

The whole family.

unable to see what is ahead. But Bill has a vision; he can see for us a hope and a future just as Nicole, my nurse and friend from Yale, promised in the hospital over fifteen years ago. We still have time.

Have I grown from this experience? I can only offer that I do not long for what I have lost. I consider this a small achievement. They were things to borrow, not for a lifetime, but for a season. I do not seek to find them again. Instead I seek what cannot be taken from me, the pleasure of seeing my daughters in their youthful beauty, the smell of the air after a good rain, and this time I share with Bill. There is no part of my life I would alter if it meant Bill was not a part of it, yet I envy those who have love and have not had to lose. And I even envy us, because for a moment we did have it all.

Epilogue

My father died on April 20, 2016. The reality of those words has not yet sunk in. I miss him every day. He never read my book, but knew every word. We travelled to Chicago for his 83th birthday, and it became our goodbye. Bill joined me along with Anna and Georgia, who was nearly three when she met her grandfather for the first—and last—time. Dad did not have to meet her in person to be bonded to her because he was, even before she was born. The closeness he shares with people does not have to be confirmed with physical time together. This occasion was me wanting him to see how God had once again blessed us. Georgia knew him immediately, "Papa," she said. "Yes Georgia, that is your Papa, doesn't he look exactly like his picture?" She smiled at him, and he beamed.

When it was time to leave, I turned to look at him one last time. He sat on the end of his bed in a white t-shirt and jeans. Every part of his body reflected its age, except for his face—he still looked as I had always known him, with a smile in his eyes.

He gave me a wink and nod, smiled, and then quietly said, "Carry on." He believed that I could.

Since his funeral, not a day has passed when I don't ask myself, "What would Dad do?" or "What would he say?" I'd sought his counsel for so long and about issues that remain unresolved. Now I must rely upon my memories, and myself. Thankfully, Dad left me with more than words, but his example. I know what he would do. He would listen more and talk less; he would offer his wisdom without judgment; and he would love with all of his strength. He believed in love as a cure, and then more love. Our time together always left me better, even when nothing tangible changed. As I looked at him in the casket, he did not seem gone—I felt him smiling at me. "Dad, come back," I whispered. "I never want to let you go." I miss his commentary, his encouraging voice, and his affirmation.

Dad was very much like the peasant character in Tolstoy's *War and Peace*, whom the principal character, Pierre, meets in prison and describes as having grasped the secret of living: "He took pleasure in the good and endured the suffering cheerfully." Dad suffered at the end. I'm sure of it. His toes were blackened from lack of blood flow. His tendons were exposed, but he was unwaveringly happy. He never complained about his pain to me. Every call began with, "Oh Annette, I am *so* pleased to hear your voice." He was my father, first and foremost; the dear, sweet man who always expressed that my life, my existence, mattered. I found it remarkable to meet so many people—strangers to me—who shared stories of what Dad had meant to them. One young woman told me, "Your father always made me feel special. He listened to me." I found it hard to fathom he could give so much to so many people. Wasn't he saving all of that encouragement for *my* phone calls? But no, he wanted to bring good to anyone in his presence. While I continue to struggle with doubt, there's no way to believe that he could sustain such charity without God. That level of love, should it come solely from one's self, would deplete us, yet his source was constant because it was also eternal, it just had to be. As he grew in faith, he became a vessel of love, not that he was perfect, but closer than anyone I have known.

Dad always said our last and greatest freedom was to choose our own attitude. There is no way I can know if my experiences of struggle have left me better, but I *have* grown. I kept the promise made to Bill on our wedding day—to love no matter what comes our way, in sickness or health, for richer or poorer, good times and bad.

I notice the lines on my face where there was once smooth skin. It is futile to hold onto anything. As my father promised, things will never stay the same, and I must find the courage to move beyond the disappointments. He is there at my side. "Coward, take my coward's hand." Together, we are less afraid.

Acknowledgements

GENEROUS FRIENDS HAVE HELPED OUR family in a thousand ways.

Dr. Strittmatter, Dr. Sadowsky, Dr. Magriples, Dr. Hasapis and Dr. Flynn—you all exemplify patient care at its very best.

Teri and Nicole—thank you both for expressing the art of caring for a patient, body and soul.

My physical therapists Ralph, Pat Rummerfield, Pat Mediate, Jennifer, Robin, Andrew and Zach—I would have never achieved any use of my legs without your patience, creativity, and perseverance.

Awakenings Health Institute and especially Laura and Adam—I thought my ten year anniversary would be the end, but you showed me it was not.

Alison—your constant source of love, joy, and wisdom gave me hope.

Mary—while you lived with us, your everyday help and calm gave the family a sense of unity. We still miss you.

Father Ian, Father Les, and Father Peter—our entire journey here is a spiritual one but sometimes I lost my way. Thank you all for setting me back on the path. Your guidance and prayers lifted us during many difficult times.

Kathy Jennings—you are an inspiration to me.

Claire Jones—you are a one-of-a-kind wife, mother, and friend.

A special thank you to Dawn, Toni, Jodi, and Mary Anne—thank you for the love and laughter. A girl could not ask for truer friends.

The gang on Hemlock Hill —we had our best and happiest memories during the ten years we lived near all of you. And to all of our New Canaan friends who are important for reasons I hope they already know.

Jacki and Greg Zehner—you were light in a time of darkness. Thank you.

Melinda and Jeff—you brought us in as family. We love you.

George and Ann—if the one reason we moved into the house next door was to be your neighbors, it was all worth it. True friendship can blossom in every season. Thank you for seeing us through.

Wendy Lamb—you were the first person to believe I had the potential to write a book, thank you for the countless hours you spent reading many first drafts and for always, always encouraging me to stay with it.

Jennifer Falvey, Lee Woodruff, and Mike Lupica—you gave your time and talent to help me. I am fortunate to know each of you, and most grateful.

Don—you provided structure for my words. Were it not for your mentorship, our story would not be a book.

I am indebted to The Hastings Center, especially to Nancy Berlinger and Tom Murray for giving me a cherished opportunity to learn, grow and be part of an extraordinary group of people who are deeply passionate about our world.

Frank Roosevelt, my don at Sarah Lawrence, who changed the course of my academic career forever. How blessed I am to know you, to have learned from you, and to call you friend.

Willow Street Press—you said YES and made a dream come true.

Susan and Fiona, my fearless publisher and forgiving editor. You are both remarkably talented people who have given my work the love that it needed to grow. I am indebted to you both and deeply appreciate the thought you have given to each detail of the story.

Ellen and John—none of it has gone as we planned, and for that I can only say I am sorry, but the childhood you provided for Bill made him the man and father he is today. I am indebted to you both.

Uncle Jim, you stand alone in your capacity to love. You've said no one is like my dad, but you are.

The family I grew up in was wholly unique. You have all made me feel special and a part of something worth remembering. Love to Buzz, Tom, Bruce, Terry, Patti, Gale, Drew and Marty.

And to the great loves of my life, our five daughters: Natalie, Anna, Ingrid, Mia, and Georgia. I love you all exactly as you are. Thank you for the indescribable ways you bring joy to my heart.

Dad, you are still there for me. Thank you for instilling in me the gift of faith. Nothing in life has given me greater purpose.

And Bill, I love you with all the love I have to give. I know you have done the same. This is for us.

About the Author

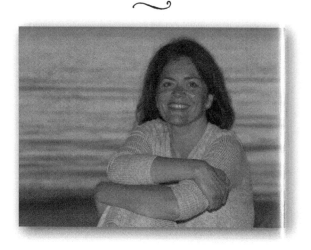

ANNETTE ROSS WAS BORN IN Chicago, graduated from Sarah Lawrence, and lives with her husband and five daughters in San Diego. This is her first book.

Photo credit: Raleigh Souther

Made in the USA
Las Vegas, NV
20 September 2021

30675239R00136